NEW DIRECTIONS IN
SEXUAL ETHICS

NEW DIRECTIONS IN SEXUAL ETHICS

MORAL THEOLOGY AND THE CHALLENGE OF AIDS

KEVIN T. KELLY

GEOFFREY
CHAPMAN

London and Washington

Geoffrey Chapman

A Cassell imprint

Wellington House, 125 Strand, London WC2R 0BB

370 Lexington Avenue, New York, NY 10017-6550

First published 1998

Reprinted 1999

British Library Cataloguing-in-Publication Data

A catalogue record for this book is available from the British Library.

ISBN 0-225-66793-2

Typeset by Keystroke, Jacaranda Lodge, Wolverhampton
Printed and bound in Great Britain by Biddles Ltd, Guildford and King's Lynn

CONTENTS

INTRODUCTION

This introduction offers a route-map for readers. It shows how the various chapters form one coherent whole, even though none of them is meant to be a thorough and exhaustive treatment of the topic they are examining.

Chapter One tells my own personal story – how the AIDS pandemic, particularly as it affects women in the developing countries, began to impinge on me and affect my thinking as a moral theologian. Behind the enormous horror of the pandemic I began to discern the voice of God calling our human family to redeem the situation by working for the radical transformation of the oppressive structures of our society which are playing such a key role in facilitating the rapid spread of HIV/AIDS in our world. The injustice of the deep-seated and far-reaching sexual and economic inequality of women is the most obvious instance of such an oppressive structure, though it is not the only one I look at. The impact this personal experience had on me has provided both the energy and direction for writing the chapters which follow.

Chapter Two examines the sociological concept of social construction. Its explores its usefulness as a tool for enabling us to understand the social and historical dimensions of ourselves as gendered sexual human persons. It helps us appreciate that such basic human realities as our gender and even our sexuality are never encountered in any pure distilled version. They are only found within a broader cultural context and will be coloured by the system of values existing within any particular culture. Hence, as actually experienced, they are to a very large extent a human artefact. As such, they should not be regarded as sacrosanct. If their current cultural expression is discerned to be contrary to human dignity in any way, we are charged with the responsibility of transforming them into a shape more in keeping with our God-given human dignity. This even applies to such basic cultural institutions as heterosexuality and marriage. To the extent that, in their present form, they may embody injustice, working for their transformation is a Christian responsibility and an essential dimension of our co-operating with God's continuing creative process.

Chapter Three looks at the position of women in particular. This chapter begins by showing how a belief in the inferior status of women seems to have operated within the life and thinking of the Church over many centuries. It then looks at how this unacceptable situation is beginning to change and sees many hopeful signs within the Roman Catholic Church itself. Of special note are some recent statements by Pope John Paul II in which he strongly defends the full and equal dignity of women and the need for this to be given practical implementation at all levels of Church and society. The chapter then builds on the previous chapter's insistence that the gender differentiation between men and women is, for the most part, socially constructed and thus open to a socially transforming reconstruction. In the light of this, the notion of an 'ontological complementarity' between men and women, a notion strongly supported by Pope John Paul II, is examined critically in the light of women's experience and also in its implications for the debate about the ordination of women. The underlying motif of this chapter is that, if our understanding of the man–woman relationship is out of kilter, our sexual ethics is bound to be at least inadequate, if not misguided. The chapter closes by suggesting that perhaps a top priority for the Church today is to support women in their efforts to free themselves from or at least radically transform any cultural institutions, including marriage, which effectively deny their equal dignity as human persons. That is why it even suggests that, if the Church is to be faithful to the demands of the Gospel, it needs to be pro-women before it is pro-marriage.

In the fourth chapter a concern for reducing the spread of HIV leads naturally into an examination of the issue of gay and lesbian relationships. Since one way the spread of the virus can be facilitated is by genital sexual contact with many partners, the conclusion would seem to follow that, within the gay and lesbian communities, one of the most effective ways to reduce the spread of the virus would be for gays and lesbians to have faithful, permanent relationships with only one partner. Yet this seems to be anathema to the official position of many Christian Churches and to many individual Christians. The chapter notes how this anti-gay and lesbian gut-reaction has been challenged in many cases by the love and care shown in many gay relationships and particularly when one partner is dying of an AIDS-related illness. It also notes how the negative position on gay and lesbian relationships in many Churches has been based on a combination of two objections: it is 'against nature' and it is 'against the Bible'. In the course of examining these two objections, the issue of social construction arises once again. The motif underlying this chapter is the belief that the Gospel must be 'good news' for gays and lesbians and that this is not the case with the present teaching of many Christian Churches. A sexual ethics which is able to be 'good news' for gays and lesbians should also be 'good news' for heterosexuals too. This is because its primary focus will be the relationship dimension of our being human persons and the potentiality of our sexuality to express interpersonal love between faithful and committed partners.

Chapter Five tries to listen to what the Churches have been saying about sexual ethics during the past century. If we are to listen to the living voice of Christian tradition, we should expect to find it somewhere in this conversation within and between the Churches. The chapter notes how there is a widening of the agenda for this conversation over the years. Advances in birth control make it possible for couples to make love without fear of having any unwanted children. This possibility begins to put the focus on how the procreational dimension of marriage fits in with the relational dimension. There is a gradual move away from seeing procreation as the primary end of marriage. Instead marriage is seen to be about the couple's love for each other. Any children to the marriage are the 'fruit' of their love rather than the *raison d'être* of their marriage. Once this relationship dimension comes to the fore, other questions quickly come on the agenda. If marriage is fundamentally about the couple's relationship, what about when their relationship dies and there is nothing left between them? So the question of marriage breakdown and remarriage after divorce comes on to the agenda. Moreover, the increasing emphasis in the Churches on the centrality of relationship and the importance of the sexual expression of this relationship in the context of interpersonal Christian love prompts gay and lesbian Christians to challenge their Churches to face up to the phenomenon of same-sex love. If it is true that they are capable of loving and faithful relationships, why should the Churches condemn the partnership of gays and lesbians? Stress on the quality of relationships as a basic criterion for sexual ethics means that still further issues begin to come on to the agenda. The basic motif behind this chapter is a belief that somewhere in this (at times) heated and confusing dialogue the voice of God's Spirit is making itself heard. Hence, this tries to be very much a 'listening' chapter. That is why, as far as is feasible, the reader is given a chance to read some of the more significant passages from the documents of the various Churches.

Chapter Six argues that there are at least six ways in which a transformed Christian sexual ethics must adopt a positive stance before life. It must be (1) *pro person*, and specifically *pro-women*; (2) *pro-freedom*; (3) *pro-relationship* and *pro-love*; (4) *pro-body*, *pro-sex* and *pro-joy*; (5) *pro-life*; and (6) *pro-respect for personal conscience*.

Paradoxically, I suspect that this chapter is the least important one in the book. There are many people far more expert and competent than I am in the specific field of sexual ethics. Returning to the conversation image employed in Chapter Five, I offer this chapter as a very modest contribution to the conversation. In my book *New Directions in Moral Theology* (London, Geoffrey Chapman, 1992, p. viii), I asked the reader to imagine the words 'I may be wrong but . . . ' as being written at the top of every page. I feel that to be particularly necessary in the case of this chapter.

Despite that, I remain strongly committed to the three points which form the major thrust of this book: – (1) the Church is not able to shoulder its important responsibility in playing a major role in responding to the challenge of the HIV/AIDS pandemic if its sexual ethics is inadequate and unconvincing; (2) as long as the Church fails to take comprehensively on board the full and equal dignity of women, it will fail to give women the help and support they need in their fight for survival against HIV/AIDS since they will find the Church's sexual ethics to be unconvincing and inadequate to their real needs; and (3) as long as the Gospel does not come over as 'good news' for gays and lesbians (and that requires a reappraisal of our sexual ethics), the Church will be failing in its God-given mission to gays and lesbians in this 'time of AIDS'.

Roman Catholic moral theology is often accused of equating sex with sin. In Chapter Seven I look at how sin would feature in a transformed Christian sexual ethics. Since we are dealing with a person-centred sexual ethics, the presence of sin will be discerned where the good of human persons is being denied or violated. Sexual sin is where this occurs in the sexual sphere, whether at an individual or social level. I argue that patriarchy can rightly be described as a 'structural' sexual sin and I explore whether the Church shares responsibility through colluding in it. The chapter ends by facing the question, 'Is trivial, uncommitted sex right or wrong?' as an example of how a person-centred sexual ethics would respond to the usual 'Is it a sin to . . . ?' questions.

Chapter Eight focuses on 'living positively in a time of AIDS'. After drawing inspiration from Uganda it asks the question: Is the Church living positively with AIDS? Its yes/no answer includes a discussion of the ethics of compulsory HIV testing for future priests and religious and also of condom-use as a component in HIV-prevention programmes. The Epilogue picks up on the words of Professor Richard Parker to the 1996 Vancouver International Aids Conference that this 'time of Aids' can be a 'time of grace'.

I cannot end this Introduction without making some attempt to thank the many people who have helped and encouraged me in the writing of this book. The list of those I would like to thank by name is impossibly long and spans many continents. Top of the list must come Dr Maura O'Donohue MMM. Without her encouragement, inspiration, and professional knowledge and experience I would never have dared to attempt this book. Her field reports from various parts of the world, along with those of Ann Smith and Jim Simmons, have helped to keep me in touch with the tragic reality of HIV/AIDS in the developing countries. The other members of the CAFOD AIDS Section and its AIDS Committee, chaired by Dr Mary McHugh, have been a further source of inspiration to me. I owe a special debt of gratitude to my fellow moral theologian, Dr Linda Hogan, who, despite enormous pressures on her own time, was always willing to read and comment on any drafts I sent her. Dr Julie Scott from the Sociology Department here at Liverpool Hope University College made some very helpful comments on Chapter Two, as did Jane McGinley SND. I am grateful to have been able to share a draft version of parts of Chapters Two and Six with fellow members of the Association of Teachers of Moral Theology. Their encouragement and comments were very helpful. Martin Pendergast of Catholic AIDS Link and Dr Elizabeth Stuart of the University of Glamorgan also helped me with their comments on Chapter Four, and Elizabeth Rees kindly read and commented on the whole final draft. Further afield, I would like to express my thanks to Dr Jon Fuller SJ who helped me in more ways than he realizes and also to Bob Vitillo for his inspiring commitment and wealth of wisdom and experience. Pat Doyle too, has helped with his continuing encouragement and offered some valuable observations on an early draft. I am grateful to Christopher O'Hare and Channel Four for permission to use material from the documentary *Better Dead than Gay*. I am also indebted to all the writers from whose works I quote. I thank them all for their contributions to the ongoing conversation which, I believe, is so essential to contemporary moral theology.

It would have been unthinkable for me to write about AIDS in the developing countries without some first-hand experience, however brief, of what the AIDS pandemic means on the ground. I am grateful to friends in Uganda, Thailand and the Philippines for making that experience possible for me: in Uganda, the Medical Missionaries of Mary and their co-workers at Kitovu Hospital in Masaka, especially Sisters Ursula Sharp and Kay Lawlor; Noerine Kaleeba and her remarkable TASO organization, Sister Miriam Duggan and her co-workers at Kamwokya and the Nsambya Hospital in Kampala; in Thailand, Sister Michelle and her Fountain of Life Centre, Pattaya for a mind-blowing exposure experience, Usanee Nansilp for making my visit to Bangkok so fruitful and enjoyable, Fr Dan Boyd MM at Welcome House, Fr Giovanni Contarin and his Camillian AIDS Relief Centre staff, Fr Antonio Egiguren OFM at the AIDS Hospice in Lamlukka, Sumitra Phongsathorn for inviting me to the Women's Circle at Mater Dei College in Bangkok, Sister Meg Gallagher MM, and especially Jean Barry SJ and his Jesuit community for their hospitality; in the Philippines, Mgr Francisco Tantoco and Sister Julma Neo for arranging my visit and the Caritas AIDS staff (Sister Oneng Mendoza, Geline Sucgang, Kyara Cruza and Marina Zamora) for sharing their very helpful experience with me, Fr Shay Cullen SSC for a most instructive overnight stay at his Preda Foundation in Olongapo City, Jomar Fleras of Reach Out, Dr Ofelia T. Monzon, Director of the AIDS Research Group in the Research Institute for Tropical Medicine, Alabbang, Dr Evelyn Grace Gacad, Head of the National AIDS–STD Prevention Programme at the Department of Health, Aida F. Santos at Wedpro, Sharon Cabusao at Gabriela, Marianna Balquidra of Remedios and, above all, Fr Thomas O'Grady SSC and his colleagues for making me so much at home during my stay in Manila. I am also most grateful to the Trust whose generous grant made these visits possible as well as funding other aspects of my research. Being based in a lively inner-city parish in Liverpool, I would never have found the time to write up my research had it not been for Professor Simon Lee, Rector of Liverpool Hope University College, offering me a part-time Research Fellowship and so enabling me to write in a very congenial setting and among friendly and supportive colleagues. Gillian Paterson of Geoffrey Chapman has been a patient and understanding editor in the face of frustrating delays. She has also helped me by her friendly encouragement and inspired me by her own fine book dealing with similar issues, *Love in a Time of AIDS: Women, Health and the Challenge of HIV* (Geneva, WCC Publications and New York, Orbis, 1996). Finally, I am particularly grateful to Jim Dunne, Fr Peter Sibert and the parishioners of Our Lady's, Eldon St, for their patience and understanding while I have been writing this book. There are many other people I would like to name but space is limited. I feel sure they know how grateful I am to them too.

To thank people for their help in the writing of a book is not to burden them with any responsibility for its many failings and shortcomings. That responsibility is mine alone. Though I know I will not have done justice to the rich experience and wisdom they have shared with me, I hope that the pages which follow go some little way to repaying my debt of gratitude to them. I also hope that the many defects and inadequacies in the book will not distract readers from hearing its main message loud and clear. That is that we are living in a 'time of AIDS' and that, if we respond positively and creatively to its challenge, we may be able to turn a major human tragedy into a moment of grace for our human family.

Kevin T. Kelly
Liverpool Hope University College
June 1997

1

HEARING THE CHALLENGE OF THE AIDS PANDEMIC:

A MORAL THEOLOGIAN TELLS HIS STORY

I had just returned from spending three weeks in Uganda to gain some first-hand experience of the reality of HIV/AIDS in the developing world. It had been a privileged, though very disturbing, experience and had made a deep impact on me. After a good night's sleep to get over my jet-lag, I was sitting in the chapel in the Little Company of Mary house in Ealing, thinking about the experience of the past three weeks – a kind of debriefing prayer session. Four words were uppermost in my mind as I sat there – 'poverty', 'women', 'sexuality' and 'limitations'. These seemed to sum up the challenge of what I had experienced in Uganda. I was also thinking about the readings for the Mass that morning. They were on the theme of speaking the word of God with integrity and how this can create division and even bring suffering and persecution! It was while all this was going on in my mind that the idea of writing this book came to me.

Later that morning I was due to have a session with Ruth McCurry, from Geoffrey Chapman, to explore the possibility of my writing a book on contemporary moral problems. One of the contemporary issues I was intending to cover was the AIDS pandemic and its ethical dimensions. However, in my debriefing session in the chapel the idea began to form in my mind that perhaps, given my gifts, experience and limitations, the book should be totally devoted to this topic. Moreover, it should not be a purely academic study. Rather it should be a Church-challenging and pastorally helpful study which would be supportive of people committed to working in the AIDS field. It would need to be written at a fairly popular level since part of its purpose would be to heighten awareness among people at large and encourage them to take this issue on board. However, at the same time it would need to be academically sound since it would be challenging some of the cultural and Church presuppositions and power-structures which seem to be part of the problem.

One of my companions on my visit to Uganda was Dr Maura O'Donohue, a Medical Missionary of Mary sister who worked in Ethiopia during the worst famine years. From 1988 until February 1997, Maura headed the AIDS section at CAFOD (Catholic Agency For Overseas Development). The AIDS pandemic had come on CAFOD's agenda because it was beginning to have a catastrophic impact on development policies in the developing world. Most of the people dying were young adults on whom the development of a country depended so much. For some time Maura had been challenging me (and other moral theologians) to face up to a number of key ethical issues being unearthed by the AIDS pandemic. Through her I was invited to become a member of the CAFOD AIDS committee. That was my first real exposure to the enormity of the HIV/AIDS pandemic and its increasing threat to many developing countries. My Uganda exposure experience was also shared with Dr Mary McHugh, chair of the CAFOD AIDS committee. CAFOD was keen that we should both be better equipped for our work on the committee.

Uganda was chosen for our 'exposure' visit since the HIV/AIDS pandemic has reached catastrophic proportions in that beautiful but long-suffering country. According to a 1996 CAFOD report, 'in a population of 18 million it is estimated that there are 1.9 million people infected with HIV'. However, Uganda is only the tip of the HIV/AIDS iceberg (a curiously apt image, remembering Britain's first introduction to AIDS on television!). The mid-1996 world figures for HIV/AIDS infection are 21.8 million, of whom 94 per cent are in developing countries. Most of these live in sub-Saharan Africa and South and South-East Asia. At present, the pandemic in South and South-East Asia may be growing at a pace reminiscent of sub-Saharan Africa in the early 1980s, but may have an even greater potential for spread, given the adult population of nearly 1 billion people as compared with 225 million in sub-Saharan Africa. It is esimated that the number of those infected with HIV in Asia will rise from 3.5 million in 1996 to 12 million by the year 2000. The vast majority of these are in India and Thailand. Moreover, it is now estimated that at least 75 per cent of cumulative HIV infections in adults have been transmitted through heterosexual intercourse.

It would be misleading to give the impression that the HIV/AIDS pandemic is occurring only in the developing world. That is not so. This is brought out in an unpublished letter to *The Tablet*, written by

Martin Pendergast, convener of CAL (Catholic Aids Link) and for many years Health Service Commissioner of HIV, Sexual Health and Drug Misuse services in North East London. Speaking from a wealth of experience in the United Kingdom, Martin challenges an editorial in *The Tablet* (13 May 1995) seeming to imply that HIV/AIDS is no longer a major issue of concern in the UK:

> The gist of your argument seems to suggest that the front line of HIV/AIDS is 'over there', wherever 'there' happens to be. Certainly, the impact is catastrophic in the developing world . . . The UK's relative success in holding HIV and AIDS incidence at lower levels than many Western European countries with large Catholic populations has been due to a sustained, integrated prevention, diagnostic, treatment and support programme over the past decade, underpinned by a high degree of confidentiality. Those of us who work together to stem this pandemic often feel like Canutes. It does not help to be told, even by implication, that the front line is elsewhere. The very nature of a pandemic is that it is here, and here, and here. This does not mean accepting an inevitable tide of further transmission and illness. Rather it involves discovering and developing ways of responding to new needs in different populations. Sadly, many parts of the Church so often speak and act as if they and the epidemic are in very different places.

I have tried to keep Martin's warning in mind throughout this book. Nevertheless, as the statistics already quoted clearly demonstrate, it cannot be denied that the pandemic has been having an enormous impact on many developing countries. This was initially the case in sub-Saharan Africa. However, more recently the HIV virus seems to be spreading rapidly in India, Asia and Latin America. In many of these cultures women, and often their children, become infected with HIV mainly because of their sexual, social and economic subordination. Preventive work based solely on change in sexual behaviour is doomed to failure. Change has to occur at a deeper social level.

I soon began to see what had become obvious to Sister Maura and her AIDS co-workers at CAFOD, namely, that injustice against women in its different manifestations is a major underlying factor in the rapid spread of HIV/AIDS in developing countries. Even at this early stage it is worth spelling this out in more detail.

WOMEN AND HIV/AIDS

In 1994 a paper entitled *Women and AIDS* was published jointly by the World Health Organization and the United Nations' Development Programme in consultation with the UN Division for the Advancement of Women. In its initial summary the report presents a very disturbing picture of the rapid spread of HIV infection among women, mainly in the developing countries:

> From being almost absent from the AIDS epidemic in the 1980s, women infected with HIV now number more than six million – with another one million women becoming infected this year. By the year 2000, over 13 million women will have been infected and 4 million of them will have died.

Although HIV infects both men and women, it seems that it is now increasingly affecting women in a disproportionate manner. The above report points out that this is due to three principal factors – the sexual subordination of women, their economic subordination and their special vulnerability due to the specific nature of female biology.

The first two of these factors, the sexual and economic subordination of women, are rooted in the denial of the full and equal dignity of women. Among the more specific ways in which these two factors actually contribute to the rapid spread of HIV/AIDS the following would seem to be most common and the most influential.

1. 'Double-standard morality'

In many cultures it is assumed that men are not bound by the same standards of morality as women. Women are expected to be virgins when they come to be married and, once married, they must be faithful to their husbands. Men, on the other hand, are expected to be sexually experienced when they approach marriage. This experience comes from their visiting prostitutes, a practice which is regarded as fairly normal and acceptable for many young men. As mentioned in one of my diary entries later in this chapter, in some places it is even one of the elements built into a stag party or its equivalent before marriage. After marriage, if the husband begins to tire of his wife, it is common for him either to seek comfort from prostitutes or to have a 'minor wife', with or without the consent of his first wife. No such licence is permitted to his wife. As a woman she must remain faithful to her husband. Because her economic and social security may be entirely dependent on him, she may find it less threatening to keep quiet and not complain, rather than challenge her husband and risk his leaving her or putting her out.

The practical effect of this double morality with regard to women and AIDS is that, in a country where HIV is spreading within the heterosexual population, it is very possible that a woman living in accord with an ethical standard of virginity before marriage and complete fidelity within marriage will still find herself infected with the virus by her husband. Possibly the first indication she will have of her infection will be the tragic news that her child has been born with the virus. This news is shattering at a whole variety of levels. Her child's life will almost certainly be short and painful. Her own health and life expectancy is seriously threatened, as is that of her husband. The future of her other children is now put at risk, due to the likelihood of their losing both their parents. And her husband's infidelity to her is now confirmed. Prior to the news of her child's infection, for her to suggest to her husband that they should practise 'safer sex' in order to safeguard her own health as well for the sake of her children would probably be unthinkable. It would implicitly be challenging her husband's fidelity and it would be assuming an equality in sexual bargaining power which is denied her by the 'double-standard morality' ethos.

2. Use of younger girls for 'safe' sex

This 'double-standard morality' which accepts more permissive sexual behaviour by men implies that many men are involved in multi-partner sexual activity. This in itself is high-risk behaviour in terms of HIV/ AIDS. However, some men who think they may not be infected with the virus are now tending to approach younger girls on the assumption that they will be virgins and so will not be infected themselves. For a variety of reasons these girls may be under great pressure to accede to their requests. They might be seen by their parents as a good source of income for the family since their education is viewed as of lesser importance than that of their brothers. Or perhaps their parents have already died of AIDS and they have to carry responsibility for their orphan-headed family. A 'sugar daddy' can be a god-send for a young girl in such a plight. Even if the young girl is at school, acceding to her male teacher's request might be the only way she can get the required pass to continue her education. A similar scenario is becoming more common within the sex industry. Young 'virgins' are in great demand because of their providing an opportunity of safe sex for their male clients. It is reported from certain parts of Burma, for instance, that, unlike the Chinese, parents are rejoicing over the birth of a girl baby. She will be a good source of income when she is old enough to be sold to a brothel in Thailand! All these scenarios constitute ways in which these young women are likely to become infected with HIV by the people abusing and exploiting them. Moreover, the risk is all the greater due to the fact that, biologically, women are more vulnerable to HIV infection than men. That is particularly true of young girls since their immature cervix and relatively low mucus production presents less of a barrier to HIV.

3. Sexual subordination of women and the sex industry

The sexual subordination of women makes the sex industry more socially acceptable, even though this does not imply that women engaged in the sex industry are given any social respect. This again is where the double standard operates. It is acceptable for men to be customers ('men will be men') and to buy the services of the women involved. But the prostitutes themselves are said to be living on 'immoral earnings' and, in some countries, are even criminalized.

Although prostitutes are often blamed for the spread of HIV/AIDS, they themselves will almost invariably have been infected by their male clients. For the most part, they will rarely be in a position to be able to insist on the use of condoms by their male clients. Consequently, because their trade involves them necessarily in multi-partner sex and because the risk for them is magnified by their biology as (young) women, they are very much at risk of HIV infection. The tragedy is that many of them will have come into the sex industry out of sheer poverty or at least as the only way they can generate sufficient income to care for their dependants. In many cultures it is the girls in the family who are expected to look after their parents and younger siblings. This burden is further aggravated by the likelihood that they may also have children of their own. When a woman labouring under such heavy pressures discovers that she is HIV positive, she finds herself in a Catch 22 situation. Naturally, faced with the possibility of her dying in the not-too-distant future, her prime concern will be for her children and dependants and how to make provision for them while the opportunity is still open to her. Hence, she might well keep secret the fact that she is infected so that she is able to continue operating for as long as possible.

4. Female genital mutilation and other cultural practices affecting women

At the end of her novel, *Possessing the Secret of Joy* (London, Vintage, 1993), Alice Walker mentions that it is estimated that 'from ninety to one hundred million women and girls living today in African, Far Eastern and Middle Eastern countries have been genitally mutilated' (p. 266). I am told that female genital mutilation as practised in some parts of Africa yields a total of ten million new cases of mutilation each year! This practice leaves women, especially young women, more at risk of HIV infection due to a number of reasons, the main one being the fact that it leaves them with permanent scar tissues which are open to abrasions in the course of sexual activity.

Cultural practices which involve multi-partner sex also increase the risk of HIV infection. In some cultures it is still acceptable for a husband to 'lend' his wife to a guest as a mark of respect, although, thankfully, this practice seems to be dying out. Another 'traditional' custom still found in some countries is wife inheritance in which a wife is 'inherited' by her husband's male next of kin. In some cultures the law restricts property ownership and inheritance to men. This only reinforces women's economic dependence on male relatives and can leave them defenceless in the face of sexual practices which can put them at risk of Sexually Transmitted Diseases (STDs) and HIV infection. Similarly, laws governing marriage, divorce and child custody can prevent women leaving a relationship in which they or their children are being sexually abused and thus exposed to the risk of HIV infection.

In most cultures, it is women who are left to bear the burden of caring for any family members who develop AIDS. Often they themselves may also be HIV infected. When there is no financial support and little support from the wider community, this leaves the women carers very vulnerable, since they may be labouring under enormous psychological and emotional pressures as they watch their loved ones dying and are fearful for the future, both for themselves and for the family. Where AIDS is rife, they may also have to carry the additional burden of caring for the orphaned children of dead relatives. Their desperate situation can obviously leave them vulnerable to men who are willing to offer economic help in return for sexual favours. Once again this is a dangerous scenario in terms of the spread of HIV/AIDS.

5. Low priority given to women's education

Girls are expected to look after the home and care for their ailing parents. Hence, they are frequently denied the possibility of a full education. This deprives them of learning to look critically at their own culture and judge whether certain tribal customs violate their true dignity as women. Hence, they are more likely to accept their sexual, social and economic subordination simply as part of their lot as women. And even when a girl gets the chance of a full education, she may be forced to have sex with her male teacher or educational official in order to get a credit or to gain entrance into college.

6. Migration

Frequently, husbands, forced to work away from home, will have few qualms about going with prostitutes while they are away or even having a more stable relationship with a woman in the locality in which they are working. This increases the possibility of husbands bringing back HIV infection to their faithful wives. Increasingly, too, in some economies in the developing world, women are finding that they need to go abroad as migrant workers in order to support their families or to attain sufficient economic independence to be able to set up home on their own. However, such women may find themselves subject to a system of sexual barter if they are to be able to obtain employment or continue in it. Sexual favours might also be asked in exchange for entry or residence permits, or in order to get transport to their employment.

THE 'PRO-WOMEN' CHALLENGE TO THE CHURCH AND TO CHRISTIAN SEXUAL ETHICS

Although the examples given above may not be found everywhere in the developing world, my own listening to women in Uganda, Thailand and the Philippines has convinced me that they are disturbingly widespread. A similar picture emerges in CAFOD reports of visits to many developing countries and in other first-hand accounts, both written and oral, I have been given of the situation of women in these lands.

In the light of the picture presented above, it would seem unrealistic and even harmful to suggest that the only real solution to the HIV/AIDS pandemic lies in the traditional 'faithful to one partner' sexual ethic. That offers no help to many women. For them, what is lacking is the very foundation without which such a sexual ethic is virtually meaningless. As long as their full and equal dignity is not accepted in theory and in practice, many of the norms of this traditional sexual ethic are likely to work against the well-being of these women and may even prove to be the occasion of their becoming infected by HIV.

It would seem obvious that there will be no substantial alleviation of the plight of women oppressed in these various ways until there is a cultural shift to accepting the full dignity of women and adapting cultural norms so that the relationships of women and men are able to be lived out in true equality and mutuality. I am very conscious that such a statement from a Christian theologian in the West can smack of cultural and religious imperialism. Criticism of any culture tends to be more credible if it comes from within that culture. That is why I believe that, if the Church is to respond to the serious moral imperative of working for the cultural integration of the full and equal dignity of women, it can best, and perhaps only, do this by giving all the support it can to women and women's movements within that particular culture who are working to bring about such an integration. Nevertheless, because power in the Church as presently constituted is almost exclusively wielded by men, the women and women's groups mentioned above may well have experienced the Church itself as part of the injustice they are trying to overcome. Where this is the case, the Church must face up to its own internal need for conversion by listening humbly to the experience of these women as they tell it themselves. In this connection, the justice dimension of sexual ethics must be taken on board by the Church. An awareness of the plight of women suffering sexual exploitation or trapped in the sex industry highlights this justice dimension. However, the Church must accept that it has implications for the entire field of sexual ethics. For instance, it would be a much more credible witness to the Gospel if the Church was renowned for its opposition to female genital mutilation rather than for its opposition to the use of condoms.

This brings up an even more fundamental point. In the light of the serious injustice suffered by so many women in the sexual sphere, it would seem that at this point in history a Christian sexual ethic should be 'pro-women' before it is 'pro-marriage'; Adapting the words of Jesus, this means recognizing that marriage is made for women, not women for marriage. Of course, it could be objected that women are not the only persons whose well-being is involved in marriage. That is true. In its pristine form the principle should read: marriage is made for persons, not persons for marriage. However, the AIDS pandemic is making us aware that the persons whose well-being may be least protected within the institution of marriage are women – particularly wives, but also daughters. This has been true over many centuries but, in our 'time of AIDS' the consequences of this injustice have become even more horrendous.

Today women, and men too, are becoming more aware of this institutionalized injustice. In fact, during the International Women's Year in 1975, Paul VI described this emerging consciousness among women of their full dignity as human persons as one of the 'signs of the times'. By his deliberate choice of this phrase, given special significance by John XXIII, he seemed to be implying that God was revealing to the Church a new dimension of our understanding of the Gospel message of liberation through this worldwide phenomenon of growing awareness on the part of women. This 'sign of the times' is why, in our age, the principle, 'marriage is made for persons', directs our attention particularly to the plight of the many women for whom marriage offers the prospect of oppression rather than of liberation and fulfilment. This same principle also challenges any culture where the very institution of marriage itself, in its current form, contradicts the respect owed to women in view of their full and equal human dignity. The inculturation of the Gospel in such a culture must necessarily be subversive of the institution of marriage as it exists in that culture. As already mentioned, this subversion will probably only be brought about through the heroic opposition of women within that culture who have a critical awareness of the inhumanity of the institution of marriage in their society.

However, the sexual and economic subordination of women is not restricted to the developing world. It is still experienced by many women in the West, though perhaps with less severe consequences than in many developing countries. Moreover, as we shall see in Chapter Three, a similar patriarchal approach to women also operates in the Church at large and perhaps most strikingly within the Roman Catholic Church. Moreover, this is not merely a brief aberration within the history of the Christian community. It has been a constant in Christian thought and practice from the earliest centuries, even though Christian feminist writers are now reclaiming the strands of an alternative and more enlightened tradition which has struggled to co-exist under the prevailing patriarchal ideology. However, the dominant mind-set right from the very early days in the Church has taken for granted the inferiority of women.

WIDENING THE AGENDA: THE NEED FOR A RENEWED SEXUAL ETHICS

While I was still early in the process of absorbing all this, CAFOD invited me to attend a meeting of English-speaking moral theologians in New York. In a paper I gave to initiate one of the discussions, I stated that one major challenge of the HIV/AIDS pandemic to the Churches and to moral theologians concerned the need to develop a more satisfactory sexual ethic. I suggested that such a sexual ethic would need to be constructed along the following lines:

1. It would need to be a sexual ethic which makes faithful sexual loving *attractive* to people and is based on values accessible to the thinking of ordinary men and women. If such a sexual ethic could be articulated in sufficiently positive language, it might help in limiting sexual intercourse to faithful sexual relationships. This would not be due to any fear of AIDS, nor because constrained by any external pressure from Church teaching, but because of the attraction of such a life-style if it is seen to be the way to achieve the greatest happiness as sexual persons.

2. It would also need to be a sexual ethic which acknowledges that faithful sexual loving is a desirable and good pattern of life for homosexual persons (linked to the need for self-acceptance and a sense of self-worth which features so strongly in 'gay spirituality'). Such a sexual ethic could give an attractive alternative to multi-partner and temporary relationships. Once again the drawing power of such an ethic would not lie in any fear of AIDS but would flow from the recognition that such loving and faithful relationships are good and desirable. The affirmation by the Church of the goodness and desirability of such loving and faithful relationships could be a support and encouragement to homosexual persons striving to achieve them.

I finished my contribution by insisting that a world 'living positively with AIDS' could be a very healthy world. This is because living positively with AIDS means accepting the challenge which the pandemic of AIDS is making to our world community. It is a challenge to change our ways radically on three different but closely related fronts by (1) promoting economic justice for all; (2) dismantling patriarchy; and (3) formulating a satisfactory person-respecting sexual ethic.

The first of the these three challenges does not feature largely in this book. That is not because I view it as less important but simply because the focus of this book is specifically on sexual ethics. However, it is touched on in the Epilogue in connection with Professor Richard Parker's inspirational paper to the 1996 9th International Conference on Aids in Vancouver. Even a renewed sexual ethics which incorporates respect for the full and equal dignity of women will have little effect in combating HIV/AIDS if it is not accompanied by a radical attempt to tackle the root causes, personal and structural, of poverty in our world.

After all, most of the causes I listed earlier for the rapid spread of HIV infection among women in developing countries can be linked together in some way or other under the umbrella title of the 'feminization of poverty'. It is poverty which drives many women into prostitution or, worse still, leads their parents to sell their young daughters into the sex industry. It is poverty which forces men to leave their wives and families and seek work far from home. It is poverty which causes women, even married women with children, to leave their families in order to find work abroad to support them. It is poverty which is occasioning the breakdown of many local communities and their cultures which, despite their inherent patriarchy, still have certain built-in safeguards to protect the dignity of women. It is poverty which lies behind the gross underfunding of medical services in many developing countries. In many developing countries, for instance, the health service lacks the funding to test all blood supplies used in transfusions. This means that, in practice, the right to infection-free blood is non-existent for women in these countries. This same poverty factor can also render meaningless the right of these women to adequate health care once they become HIV positive.

The more I have learned about the AIDS pandemic, the more convinced I have become that this pandemic is helping to open our eyes to some implications of the Gospel which until now have only been latent but which today are beginning to be seen as enormously important. The process of hearing these 'new, yet old' calls of the Gospel is linked to our growing awareness of certain evils which have permeated human life over the centuries and to which as Church we seem to have accommodated ourselves down the ages. Somehow the AIDS pandemic is exposing these evils in their true colours and their horror and destructiveness is becoming clear, if we only have eyes to see with.

In no way am I suggesting that AIDS had been sent by God to open our eyes to these Gospel values. That would be a blasphemous suggestion. AIDS is a human catastrophe of global magnitude and can rightly be described as one of the major evils of our day. Nevertheless, paradoxically, good can come from evil. Just as a fatal air-crash can reveal a dangerous design fault in an aircraft, so the AIDS pandemic seems to be revealing some major flaws in the social construction of man–woman gender roles, in the ethical evaluation of our sexual relationships, in our global approach to social justice, and in the way we handle the creative potential of the present moment.

As Edward Schillebeeckx reminds us, God often speaks to us through the 'contrast experience' of our inhumanity towards each other (cf. *God, the Future of Man*, London, Sheed & Ward, 1969, p. 136). The voice of God is heard in the cries of suffering caused by such inhumanity. The AIDS pandemic is making us more attentive to God's voice coming to us through the cries of women living with HIV/AIDS. The 'contrast experience' consists in the denial in practice of their full human equality and in their sexual exploitation. In the midst of the inhumanity of this situation, the cry of God's creative Spirit is heard: 'Become more truly human'. Salvation today is inextricably bound up with hearing this cry. Out of the tragedy of all the suffering and dying of AIDS can come a new step forward in the salvation of our human family. To close our ears to this is to refuse to listen to the Gospel speaking to us today.

This conviction has been with me throughout the writing of this book. That is why, when my publishers suggested the title *New Directions in Sexual Ethics*, as a link with my previous book, *New Directions in Moral Theology*, I insisted on the sub-title *Moral Theology and the Challenge of AIDS*. Although I was uneasy because the 'New Directions' title on its own seemed to promise more than I could deliver, my main worry was that such a title gave no indication that my fundamental concern in this book is with the challenge of the HIV/AIDS pandemic. The sub-title helps to keep the spotlight on the HIV/AIDS pandemic and its challenge to all of us, in the Church and in society as a whole.

LISTENING TO EXPERIENCE

To share my feeling of urgency about the need for the Church to respond adequately to the HIV/AIDS pandemic, I would like to quote a few passages from my Uganda diary. These excerpts might give readers a taste of the HIV/AIDS 'exposure' I experienced on my visit to Uganda.

The first excerpt describes a visit with one of the Home Care teams from Kitovu hospital to a little centre in the village of Kabonera in the district of Masaka:

At Kabonera everyone gathered at the house of Gerard, who is the community co-ordinator, supervising 30 community workers, all volunteers like himself. Bobo, one of the two nurses on the Home Care Team, held her clinic out of doors, round the side of Gerard's little house. It was very hot that afternoon, so we had to keep moving our chairs to stay in the shade. Each patient would sit on one side of Bobo, while I sat on the other side of her. Bobo got their permission to explain their medical records to me and also their circumstances at home.

The first to come looked a very old man but was only 52! His wife had been married before and, unknown to him, her first husband had died of AIDS. He only discovered this later when she also died of AIDS. The rest were all women, except for two children who were both brought by their sisters. All but one of the women were AIDS widows who now had AIDS themselves. One of the children was a little girl, aged 8. She looked about 3! She was born HIV+; apparently this accounted for her poor development. Her twin sister had already died of AIDS. Another woman, aged 20, was clearly very afraid. She was having constant diarrhoea. She knew that this had been the beginning of the end for many of her young friends who had died of AIDS. Another woman, aged 40, was in an advanced stage of AIDS. She had 5 children and was clearly worried about what would happen to them.

When everyone had seen either Bobo or Betty, the other nurse, and had collected their medicines from the van (and also food supplies, when needed), those who wanted to got together for a Communion service. Bobo had told me that some might want to go to confession, so we agreed that the best thing would be to incorporate a General Absolution in the Communion service. I found out later that this was unheard of in Uganda! However, it seemed to make sense to the women there. It had been explained to me earlier that part of the local culture was that women are brought up from an early age to kneel before men! This is even taken to the extreme of a wife being expected to serve her husband's meal on her knees and then to eat her own meal afterwards. Some of the women are trying to change this, since it is symbolic of the inferior position of women in their culture. Since lack of true respect for women is one of the root causes affecting the spread of AIDS, our group were very alert to any signs of this in practice. For the Communion service, the women all knelt down on the bare floor, so I knelt down with them. Since they could not understand English, I got Bobo to explain that part of the rite of Absolution was my going round each of them and laying my hands on their heads. I also got her to explain that I needed forgiveness as much as they did. So I would kneel down in front of one of them and that person would need to stand up and put her hands on my head to include me in the absolution. On this occasion I knelt in front of Bobo while she gave me absolution. This was to reverse their custom and let them see a man kneeling before a woman. At the second Home Care Visit in Kitanga, I did the same thing but this time knelt in front of one of the women with AIDS.

In the jeep on the way back I was commenting on the fact that almost all the AIDS patients were youngish women who were widows. I asked Bobo whether, in view of the degrading attitude to women in their culture, the death of a husband might, paradoxically, have an element of liberation in it. She said that was not so. This was because the husband represented security both as regards finance and property. Moreover, since the tradition is that women cannot inherit property, on the death of the husband the house and the bit of land around it would automatically go to the husband's brother. It would be up to him whether he allowed the widow and her children to remain living there. Formerly, he would even inherit his brother's widow and children.

The second excerpt recounts a visit to some Orphans Projects in Rakai. That is the district worst affected by AIDS in Uganda. Of the 8,700 orphans cared for by the Kitovu Hospital Orphans Project, 4,300 of them live in Rakai district. There 75 per cent of the children of ten years and under are orphans.

Our first visit was to an orphan-headed family. The parents had died of AIDS 4 years ago. The children had been looked after by the mother's sister until she too died of AIDS. The family is headed by a young girl aged 12, who looks after her two brothers, one aged 11 and the other 9. All three are at school, their fees paid for by the Orphans Project. The project has also built them a tiny little house with a bit of ground attached for growing foodstuffs. From there we went to Kisaalizi Primary school. There are 475 children in the school (aged from 5 to 16) and 365 of them are AIDS orphans.

We next drove on a terrible road through a jungle of banana trees and finally came to a little clearing where another orphan-headed family were living. This was a family of 7 children, headed by their sister, aged 20. Their parents had died of AIDS about 3 years previously. They had then been looked after by their mother's sister. After she too died of AIDS, the eldest girl, aged 25, looked after them – and had a baby herself during this time. Then she too died of AIDS. So now the next eldest sister is in charge. The Orphans Project are helping the family reclaim some of the banana plantation which has gone wild. This will allow them to generate some income for themselves. They are also paying the eldest girl's fees to train as a teacher.

Our next visit was to another orphan family, this time looked after by their grandmother, aged 84. There were 6 children, the eldest aged 14. Their parents had died in 1990 and 1991. The Project pays the children's school fees. The granny was thrilled with our visit. She insisted on doing a 'welcome' dance inside her little house.

The main purpose of these orphans' projects is to help either guardian-headed or orphan-headed families to be able to reach a fair standard of self-reliance, even, if possible, generating their own income to cover necessities such as school fees, etc. When a young girl is head of an orphan-headed family, she is under great pressure. Poverty means that she has no money to buy things for herself, despite peer pressures from other girls at school. Hence, there is a great danger of her being exploited by older men – sexual favours for little practical gifts. This is a further reason why income-generating projects are so important.

A final excerpt contains parts of three conversations I had in Kampala:

We talked with Francis, the senior counsellor in the Home Care unit, about the danger of Western-style counselling destroying the traditional, cultural structures of elders in the local communities with all their natural wisdom and counselling skills. Francis was very alert to this danger but said that many elders lacked accurate information and knowledge about AIDS. Hence, there was a danger that they might defend negative cultural features (especially regarding women) which help in the spread of AIDS and increase the suffering of women. Also, these elders tend to be men.

Francis was also very frank about some other cultural practices which are now dying out but which were extremely oppressive of women and have certainly left their mark on the man–woman relationship there:

• a father would initiate his son's wife into sex

- lending his wife to a male guest or to one of his brothers was a natural gesture of 'hospitality' offered by a husband
- when a husband died, his brother inherited his wife.

After this, we had a most interesting conversation with two young women, Helen and Celia. They confirmed everything Francis had been saying. However, they made it clear that women were beginning to stand up against the repressive side of their culture. But they admitted that many women are still stuck in the cultural pattern of dependence, being little more than servants to the husband and all his family. They also pointed out that often men are still trapped in the cultural attitude of thinking that they are not 'worthy men' unless they have produced children. (And unless worthy men, they do not deserve a fitting family burial! I wondered about the implications of this for celibacy!) This attitude has implications for men who are HIV+. They still need to produce children and so insist on having sex with their wives. We also talked about rape and sexual violence. Helen and Celia said that because some women were beginning to refuse sex to HIV+ men, some of these men were looking for alternatives in the weaker section of the population – with a consequent increase in child sexual abuse and rape. Both Helen and Celia saw a change coming mainly through the economic independence of women, which in turn was helped by education and activities such as income-generating projects and women's self-awareness groups.

Later in the day I talked with a non-Ugandan priest about the position of priests with regard to AIDS in Uganda. I picked up the impression that AIDS was fairly widespread among the clergy and that many young priests had died from AIDS ('perhaps 25 per cent in some parts'). He also confirmed what I had heard before I came to Uganda, namely, that many priests in this and other African cultures find celibacy alien to them and are either living openly with 'wives' or else are having sexual relations with a number of women. Many seminarians too are sexually active. He even mentioned a case in which a doctor was giving a talk to seminarians about AIDS and the only question they seemed interested in was what were the safest condoms to use!

Six months after my visit to Uganda, I had the privilege of visiting Bangkok for a meeting of Asian theologians on HIV/AIDS. Afterwards, I stayed on for two extra weeks to get some personal experience of the AIDS scene in Thailand and the Philippines. I also wanted to meet some involved Catholic women's groups and listen to their views. As with my Ugandan experience, my visit to Bangkok and Manila

confirmed everything Maura O'Donohue had been saying about the
inferior status of women in society and how this was contributing to
the rapid spread of HIV/AIDS. Again, a few excerpts from the diary
of my visit might help readers share a bit of my experience. The first
gives some points from a round-table discussion with a group of women
in Bangkok:

(1) Everyone seemed to agree that the status of women in Thai
culture – and in the Church – was that of second-class persons.
Hence, they stressed that one of the main ways this could be
challenged and changed was through giving young women a
good education. The main thrust of this educational focus lies in
forming young women who will have an ability for critical analysis
so that they can evaluate the influences on their lives and so see
where change is needed and where culture needs to be challenged
and transformed. Sumitra was very strong on this point. She saw
this as the major role of a Catholic school in a Buddhist society.
I was fascinated by her emphasis, since she is the first lay head of
the major Catholic girls' school in Bangkok and at least 90 per
cent of her 1,800 pupils are Buddhist.

(2) Due to the poverty of families in the agricultural areas
where the local means of livelihood have been destroyed by the
country's economic policy, girls are having to come to the cities to
earn a living and often the only way to earn a 'living wage' is
through prostitution. Some are even sold into prostitution by their
parents and brothers. Also, many girls become prostitutes out of
a sense of duty to their family.

(3) Sumitra quoted a Christian Brother in charge of a large
Boys' School as saying that there is no point in struggling against
the cultural tide. Prostitution is simply part of the cultural scene
in Thailand. For most young men their first sexual experience will
be with a prostitute and the double standard morality practised
by men takes it for granted that married men can continue to
frequent prostitutes. As long as that remains the case, the sex
industry will continue and it will be the only source of income
for many women. Others in the group confirmed this picture of
Thai culture. It was claimed that 80 per cent of Thai men went
to prostitutes. Vichai, a young Jesuit sitting in on the meeting, told
the story of his first day at university. Apparently, the opening talk
to the freshers included the recommendation to go to a prostitute
that first evening. I remembered too that at the consultation
someone had pointed out that at the Stag Party on the eve of a
wedding the groom is expected to visit a prostitute.

(4) Also, it was stressed that the educational system has tended to form 'yes' women – and Christian education has often aggravated that tendency. Usanee said that the same was true with regard to the family. Parents want 'yes' children, especially in the case of girls. Once again the stress was on changing to a more critical approach to education. The thought struck me that, when this is seen as so crucial to the empowerment of women and so necessary in breaking the shackles of women's oppression (and therefore such a vital part of Christian education in 'a time of AIDS'), what a tragedy it is that part of officially approved Catholic formation is to inculcate a 'yes' attitude to Church authorities. This seems to contradict the heart of what the Gospel demands for today. I could not help thinking of Margaret Farley's hermeneutic principle: whatever works against the promotion of the true dignity of women cannot be a true interpretation of the Gospel or part of the work of redemption.

The second excerpt summarizes some of a conversation I was privileged to have with three highly committed Filipino women in Manila, all of them working full-time for Church agencies:

They all agreed that the inferior status of women was a major issue to be faced. It was built into Filipino culture which in turn merged with Catholic life-style here. Poorer women especially have the control of their bodies taken away from them. Poverty and the need to care for their family drives some of them into prostitution where they are treated as sex objects and have no bargaining power to protect themselves. Quite apart from prostitution, the prevailing attitude among men who are married is that they have the right to demand sex and women feel themselves obliged to give in to this. Among the poor there is a lot of physical violence and wife-beating in relationships; among the more educated the violence tends to be psychological and emotional. Although men may give the money they earn (not all of it!) to their wives for housekeeping, this does not operate on the level of a mutual partnership. It merely imposes on women the burden of having to make ends meet on inadequate means and leaves them open to blame when the money runs out. Basically, marriage is a culture of ownership. Double standards operate too. Women are expected to be virgins when they marry, whereas men are expected to have had sexual experience. Women even collude in this by seeing such prior sexual experience as something desirable in a man. Going to a prostitute tends to be seen as an acceptable way of sexual initiation for a man. Even within marriage, casual extra-marital relationships seem to be tolerated for men, but not for women.

The final 'exposure' experience I would like to share from my visit to Bangkok and Manila is a meeting with a young Filipino woman whom I will call Maria. (I have promised to respect her anonymity.) Maria herself told me her story. While still young she was raped by her father. This terrible experience left her feeling unclean and worthless and fit only for the rubbish dump. She felt she was now sub-standard. Moreover, as is usually the case with the eldest daughter, her parents expected her to be responsible for looking after her younger sisters and brothers, as well as providing for themselves. Maria felt this obligation all the more since she wanted to safeguard her young sisters from her father.

She tried a variety of jobs but the pay was never enough to support them. Eventually, like so many other girls in her situation, out of desperation she was forced into prostitution through sheer poverty. Her decision could hardly be called a free choice; it was the only way to earn enough to support her sisters. The way Maria put it to me was that she felt so worthless and unclean, she had nothing to lose by becoming a prostitute. It was all she was good for – and it would help to save her sisters. As she was saying this, I could not help thinking of the words of Jesus, 'Greater love has no one than to lay down one's life for one's friends.'

Inevitably Maria became infected with HIV. Paradoxically, this brought her into contact with a Catholic organization which made it possible for her to give up working as a prostitute. She now helps this organization with its AIDS-prevention educational work. Maria is also spending a lot of time helping men and women in the more advanced stages of full-blown AIDS. Not only is this exposing her to other infections due to her compromised immune system. It is also making her face the suffering and physical degradation that is almost certainly to be her lot too. Maria spoke very openly to me about this prospect lying ahead for her, probably in the fairly near future. She said she trusted God absolutely and knew he would be with her through whatever horrors she had to face. As she was speaking I was almost moved to tears by her deep faith and utter trust in God.

Hate the sin and love the sinner is the pastoral advice we are given. In Maria's case, that could be interpreted as meaning that we should hate Maria's sin of becoming a prostitute but love her, the sinner. I believe that would be a serious misreading of the situation. It came home to me very forcefully as I listened to Maria that she and the many other women whose story is similar to hers should in no way be regarded as sinners. They are the victims of sin. They are the victims of the sin of the men who abuse them and of the widespread sinful attitude that regards women as inferior to men, a sinful attitude shared by many in our own country and even in our own Church. It is a structural sin that I, and my fellow male clergy, collude in to a greater or lesser extent. Maria and many women like her are also victims of the institutionalized injustice of an economic system which has destroyed the livelihood of the farming communities that most of these women come from and reduced them and their families to abject poverty. The roots of that structural sin are found more in the West than in developing countries like the Philippines.

2

NEW DIRECTIONS?

WHY DO WE NEED 'NEW DIRECTIONS' IN SEXUAL ETHICS?

'New Directions' might seem a disturbing title for a book on sexual ethics. Human sexuality is as old as the human race. It would surely be the height of folly for each age to try to re-invent the wheel. Men and women, reflecting on their experience over the long course of human history, have accumulated a rich heritage of wisdom about how to live together as sexual persons. Christians, too, have brought the light of faith to this experience-based reflection and have developed their specific understanding of who they are as sexual persons and how this affects how they should live together. Furthermore, as a Roman Catholic moral theologian, I have to face the fact that over the centuries the Roman Catholic Church has developed a large body of teaching in the area of sexuality, human relationships and marriage. With such a wealth of accumulated wisdom, is it not presumptuous and foolish to suggest that as human beings and Christians we might need to explore new directions in the way we live our sexual lives? Should we not be trying to recover the old directions which have served people so well in the past?

The 'People of God' model of Church embraced by the Second Vatican Council reminds us that we are a pilgrim Church, a people on the move. We are on a journey of exodus out of unfreedom and journeying towards the freedom of the Kingdom of God. Although the way ahead is not always clear, we must keep going forward with confidence in the belief that, despite our many deviations *en route*, the Holy Spirit will continue to inspire us with a sense of direction as we move on our way through history. The one thing we must not do as the People of God is to call an end to our journey, claiming that we have reached our destination and so are now in a position to be able to settle down permanently. A pilgrim openness to new knowledge and understanding is taken for granted in one of the key documents of Vatican II, *The Church in the Modern World*:

> The experience of past centuries, the advances in the sciences and the treasures hidden in the various forms of human culture, which disclose human nature more completely and indicate new ways to the truth, are of benefit also to the church. From the beginning of its history it has learned to express Christ's message in the concepts and languages of various peoples, and it has also tried to throw light on it through the wisdom of philosophers, aiming so far as was proper to suit the gospel to the grasp of everyone as well as to the expectations of the wise . . . To develop such an exchange, especially in a time characterised by rapid change and a growing variety in ways of thought, the church has particular need of those who live in the world, whether they are believers or not, and who are familiar with its various institutions and disciplines and understand them intimately. It is for God's people as a whole, with the help of the Holy Spirit, and especially for pastors and theologians, to listen to the various voices of our day, discerning them and interpreting them, and to evaluate them in the light of the divine word, so that revealed truth can be increasingly appropriated, better understood and more suitably expressed. (n. 44, cf. also n. 58)

In the light of this 'pilgrim people' model of Church, the phrase 'new directions' in the title of a book on Christian sexual ethics should cause neither surprise nor apprehension to its Catholic or Christian readers. In fact, it is a fairly obvious kind of title for a book intended to serve the needs of a people on the move. Admittedly, 'new directions' is not the only emphasis that is appropriate. Another emphasis might be to explore the journey so far, how we have arrived at where we are and how we have coped with the uncertainties we have met *en route*. Yet another emphasis might be to examine where we are at present, appreciating the goodness of this present stage of the journey but also helping us to see more clearly why we are still far from the end of the journey.

Of course, these three emphases cannot be isolated from each other. The only way we can go forward is by moving from where we are. That has to be our starting-point. Moreover, the clues as to where we should be going have to be found in a careful examination of where we are and where we have been. We need to discern the direction forward from that of going backwards and retracing our journey. Moreover, we already have a lot of experience in path-finding. Hence, we need to make use of that experience. How we have succeeded in moving forward in the past can help us see how we should continue to move forward today. Hence, although the emphasis in this book will mainly be on 'new directions' in our exploration, the directions which served us well in the past will not be ignored and our present bearings will also be given careful consideration.

Moreover, the People of God is multi-lingual. It is made up of many voices. Although we believe that the voice of God's guiding Spirit is speaking to us in the midst of this multiplicity of sound, it may not be easy to interpret what precisely the Spirit is saying to us at this particular stage of our journey. Some voices in the People of God might seem to claim to have the last word with regard to what the Spirit is saying to us. Yet tradition would suggest that not to expect any final definitive word may often be more in keeping with God's ways with his people. Consequently, following the advice of F. R. Leavis, perhaps a more appropriate response to those whose God-given teaching role we accept and respect should be 'Yes, but . . . ' rather than *causa finita est*, there is nothing more to be said.

In the light of the above considerations, these chapters are written with a certain diffidence. I do not claim that they are a full or adequate presentation of Roman Catholic sexual ethics, still less of authoritative Roman Catholic teaching on sexual morality. They are simply a personal account of where I, a fairly run-of-the-mill Roman Catholic moral theologian, stand at this particular stage on our shared journey. As Chapter One has made abundantly clear, I feel deeply about these issues, especially in view of their practical implications for people's lives 'in a time of AIDS'. That is why I am sharing what to me makes Christian and Roman Catholic sense at this critical moment in the story of our human family. I hope it will help towards our better responding to the call of God's Spirit coming through the human tragedy of the HIV/AIDS pandemic.

A PROCESS IN WHICH CHANGE IS TRANSFORMING RATHER THAN DEFORMING

In his book *Religion and the Making of Society: Essays in Social Theology* (Cambridge University Press, 1994), pp. 37–8, Charles Davis makes the point that, while religious faith should play a revolutionary role in society since it relativizes every existing order, this does not imply that its effect needs to be destructive of what has gone before. Religious faith is concerned with transformation and renewal. It refuses to see the old as absolute and unchangeable. But likewise it refuses to see proposed changes as unambiguously good. As Karl Rahner once remarked, there comes a time when change is necessary if life is to continue. However, we are constantly tempted to justify change by painting the old as totally erroneous and devoid of value and presenting the new as beyond criticism and perfect in every way. In reality, even when the need for change is undeniable, we usually lose something good in the process and the new inevitably brings its own problems and disadvantages (cf. Karl Rahner, *Grace in Freedom*, Burns & Oates, London, 1969, pp. 40–4).

Consequently, if we are exploring new directions in sexual ethics, we need to be aware that these new directions are emerging out of a process. They are not a radical new beginning which consigns all former directions to the rubbish tip. What we should expect to find is that religious faith is continually struggling with this transformation process. And it is a struggle since there will always be those who resist change and claim that 'tradition' is absolute and unchangeable. Likewise, there will also be those who believe the old is beyond redemption and so have no patience with the process of renewal and transformation.

One reason why renewal and transformation are constantly needed is the fact that our knowledge of reality is constantly increasing and changing and this inevitably affects the way we live our lives. For instance, it makes an enormous difference if our understanding of homosexuality changes from regarding those who engage in same-sex behaviour as either deviant or sick 'heterosexual' persons to seeing them as persons whose fundamental orientation attracts them to persons of the same sex. Something similar could be said of our increased understanding of the human reproductive process and how this can be controlled by modern pharmaceutical compounds or new technology.

However, in recent years we have become more aware of a further reason for recognizing the need for renewal. The world in which we live, the social and relational structures which govern our lives and even the very language and thought patterns which enable us to think, are all, to a very large degree, a social construct. In other words, they do not come to us pre-packaged from God. They are all things which human creativity and ingenuity have helped to bring into being. To recognize that much of life is the product of a human making opens our eyes to the possibility that certain features of life which had been viewed as unchangeable are, on the contrary, open to be changed. Human beings have played a part in bringing them into being, so human beings can help to change them. It would be foolish to view this possibility as an open invitation to change everything in sight. That would be a recipe for disaster. However, it does alert us to the fact that, when we are faced with certain dehumanizing and oppressive traditions or cultural practices which we had previously regarded as unalterable, it may be within our power to eliminate them or, at least, change them for the better.

This ties in with a contemporary Christian understanding of the theology of creation. Our Christian God is not a divine clock-maker who, through an initial act of creation, sets the whole process of evolution in motion and then sits back to let it operate on its own. While the whole of creation is 'other' than God, it is also continuously held in being by God. Of course, this is not a new insight. Aquinas wrote very profoundly about the transcendence and immanence of God. Theologically, therefore, creation is not understood as some initial act of God. It is an on-going process and relationship. As such, therefore, creation is not some finished product of God which demands our respect through a kind of 'do not touch' response. Creation is on-going here and now. It is a 'doing' of God, in which human persons, as intelligent beings made in God's image, are called to play an indispensable role. What Charles Davis calls a basic trust in or love of 'Reality' should move us to play our responsible role in this process of transformation (*Religion and the Making of Society*, p. 35). This also leads us to take account of sin and human irresponsibility. The reality which comes to us largely as a social construct is both 'graced' and 'sin-affected'. In other words, the reality we receive, ourselves included, has been worked on already. It has been affected by the process of social construction. As a result, it will be to some extent both 'flawed' and 'value added'.

The important question, therefore, is not 'Why is change necessary?' but 'How can we affect and manage change so that it will be beneficial to us as human persons and to our planet at a whole?' Not all change is transformation. Some changes can be deforming rather than trans-forming. How to distinguish changes which are 'transforming' from those which are 'deforming' is where the task of religious ethics come in. I say 'religious ethics' deliberately, though I am not restricting religious ethics to Christian ethics. I agree with Davis when he says that for human rationality to survive at a deeper level than 'the efficient adaptation of means to ends' some kind of religious faith is needed. By religious faith here he means faith in the sense of 'an unrestricted openness to Reality' (*Religion and the Making of Society*, p. 37). Such faith could also be spoken of as an openness to be 'moved' to transformative action by the mystery of Reality. In more explicitly religious language, such openness could also be interpreted as a 'radical obedience' to the will of a transcendent/immanent God moving us to continue the process of creation through human agency.

UNDERSTANDING OURSELVES AS HISTORICAL, SOCIAL AND CULTURAL PERSONS

As human persons, we are social, cultural and historical beings. Even the very process of becoming ourselves as human persons has a historical and social dimension to it. Although it might appear a purely natural process, almost like our breathing in the air around us, it is not something we bring about on our own. Our natural 'inculturation' means our taking on board the wide spectrum of thought, language, custom, and so forth which constitutes what is meant by becoming a human person within the culture into which we are born.

Clearly, changes take place in cultures. This can happen through growth occurring in the self-understanding of the people in whom a culture is embodied. Hence, although our self-identity as human persons is, to a large extent, socially constructed, paradoxically, culture, which leaves its mark on us so profoundly in this way, can also be changed by us, since it is in itself humanly constructed and our human freedom plays a part in that ongoing process. Precisely because it owes its continued existence over the ages to this ongoing process of social construction, human culture is essentially historical. As historical, it is always open to further development and change, even, at times, radical change. However, that change does not happen independently of human agency. It does not occur purely by accident or as the result of some determined plan of destiny. Human beings are not unthinking automatons, passively absorbing cultural change. We are necessarily involved in the whole process. That is why it is so important that we are conscious of the cultural changes which are taking place so that we can try to make sure that they are beneficial to the good of human persons and our environment.

In speaking of culture here I mean everything which goes to make up how people in a society live and interact together, how they understand themselves and each other, what makes them tick, how they regard society itself and organize life in society, the kind of the language they use, the symbols which convey basic significance for them, and so forth. To my mind, one of the best definitions of culture is that given by Vatican II:

> The word 'culture' in its general sense indicates all those factors by which as human persons we refine and unfold our manifold spiritual and bodily qualities. It means our effort to bring the world itself under our control by our knowledge and labour. It includes the fact that by improving customs and institutions we render social life more human both within the family and in the civic community. Finally, it is a feature of culture that through the course of time human beings express, communicate, and conserve in their works great spiritual experiences and desires, so that these may be of advantage to the progress of many, even of the whole human family. (*The Church in the Modern World*, n. 53)

The notion of social construction helps us make sense of our human experience. It is a notion which could appropriately be described as 'revelatory'. It helps us to see in a new and richer light what has always been before our eyes but never before been perceived in this way. It puts into words what we have had an inkling of in our hearts. In a sense, it increases our ability to be moral agents in the social sphere since it makes us more aware of what is happening and how we can influence it.

However, some theologians are suspicious of the notion of social construction. They mistakenly interpret it as a philosophical theory based on the belief that human freedom reigns supreme and all reality is simply raw material for human freedom to fashion as it likes. John Paul II's advisers on *Veritatis Splendor* may have misinterpreted social construction in this way. Nevertheless, I can fully endorse the Pope's rejection of any approach which 'ultimately means making freedom self-defining and a phenomenon creative of itself and its values' (*Veritatis Splendor*, n. 46), while at the same time accepting the notion of social construction as a very helpful sociological tool for under-standing the historical processes we are involved in as cultural human persons.

A Christian theology of creation means that we accept the whole of reality, ourselves included, as given and gift. The task of human freedom is to become who we are and we cannot do that without continually trying to understand better who we are. This is a never-ending process. The notion of social construction helps us appreciate the social, cultural and historical dimensions of that process. It broadens our understanding of what is implied in coming to know and do God's will since it reminds us that no existing human structure can be regarded as definitive in terms of God's will. In a sense, therefore, the social process of helping to construct a culture which more fully embodies respect for all human persons can truly be spoken of as 'creating God's will'. That is simply drawing out the social implications of what the Pope calls for when he states that 'the moral life calls for that creativity and originality typical of the person, the source and cause of his own deliberate acts' (*Veritatis Splendor*, n. 40). This is very different from an extremist libertarian interpretation of human creativity rejected by the Pope.

SOCIAL CONSTRUCTION AND NATURAL LAW

The notion of social construction is a very enlightening contribution from the field of sociology. Despite some indications of a slight revival of the school of 'socio-biology' with its determinist interpretation of the findings of genetics and endocrinology, social construction theory seems to be the accepted thinking among most sociologists today, especially when it comes to understanding ourselves as sexual human persons. It seems to be generally agreed that, to a large degree, our sexuality, whether in the form of heterosexuality or homosexuality, is a social construct. In other words, our sexuality, as a human phenomenon, does not exist outside of history but can actually be influenced, modified and even changed through the interplay of various cultural variables in the course of history. If this is true, it would seem to follow that our sexual ethics needs to be open to modification and reappraisal to take account of significant changes occurring in our sexuality. That is why I look on social construction as a very important tool in a contemporary exploration of the field of sexual ethics.

The application of the notion of social construction to human sexuality might seem to be diametrically opposed to a natural law approach to morality. If change is possible in the sphere of human sexuality, it seems impossible for us to speak theologically about our sexuality being gift from God. It sounds more like the product of human manipulation – or, at least, of the vagaries of human history. That is far from being the case. In fact, very rich insights can be drawn from combining the enriched contemporary understanding of natural law with the notion of social construction. The theological concept of natural law provides a very enlightening interpretative lens for our

examination of the human reality which we have been helped to
understand better through the notion of social construction.

At the outset of its discussion of marriage and the family (n. 59),
the Second Anglican–Roman Catholic International Commission's
1994 Statement, *Life in Christ: Morals, Communion and the Church*, runs thus:

> Neither of our two traditions regards marriage as a human inven-
> tion. On the contrary, both see it as grounded by God in human
> nature and as a source of community, social order and stability.
> Nevertheless, the institution of marriage has found different
> expression in different cultures and at different times. In our own
> time, for instance, we are becoming increasingly aware that some
> forms, far from nurturing the dignity of persons, foster oppression
> and domination, especially of women.

When I read that passage, it reminded me of a piece I was asked to
write for *The Universe* some years ago as a commentary on the statement, 'The institution or custom of marriage has God for its author.'
Part of what I wrote is relevant to our exploration of how the merger
between natural law theory and the notion of social construction
can help us in our continuing quest to understand ourselves better as
God-given sexual persons:

> To say that God is the author of marriage does not commit
> us to believing that God issued some kind of formal decree
> commanding marriage to come into being. We can assume that
> men and women, by using their God-given intelligence to reflect
> on their developing experience, discovered that this was the 'good'
> way for most men and women to live together. Though it had its
> difficulties, it brought them happiness and security and provided
> a home for their children, thus enabling the human family to
> increase and grow. . . . We allow God to be author of marriage
> to the extent that we are open to discovering how best marriage
> should be lived today. We have an understanding of human
> sexuality and the generative processes that was not available to our
> ancestors. We know the way the sexual dimension of our lives has
> a crucial impact on our growth as persons right from our earliest
> years. We have a better insight into the way human relationships
> develop and the stages through which they need to pass. Our
> understanding of history and culture, too, has made us aware that
> our 20th century Western, rather romantic, image of marriage
> with its accompanying 'nuclear family' model is just one possible
> way in which the marriage relationship can be lived – and not
> necessarily the best way! . . .

There is much ambiguity about the new possibilities opening up for marriage and the new forms of committed sexual relationship which are claimed by some to be marriage without the pomp and circumstance. Contraception is not an unalloyed good – or evil. Neither is *in vitro* fertilization or other options now available. However, whether they are judged acceptable cannot depend on purely bio-logical criteria. Even our sexual biological make-up does not offer us an adequate criterion. After all, Catholic social teaching is all about our transforming primitive 'natural' life into human culture.

A Christian theology of creation, therefore, does not imply a 'hands-off' approach, as though all we had to do was to obey the Maker's instructions inscribed in nature. As Josef Fuchs remarks, all that 'nature' shows us is what God has brought into being:

> When in fact, nature-creation does speak to us, it tells us only what it is and how it functions on its own. In other words, the Creator shows us what is divinely willed to exist, and how it functions, but not how the Creator wills the human being qua person to use this existing reality. The person, created as a rational and prudent being must interpret, evaluate, and judge the realisation of nature from the moral point of view. (*Moral Demands and Personal Obligations*, Washington, Georgetown University Press, 1993, pp. 99–100)

'Nature' does not carry moral imperatives inscribed within it. Moral imperatives are the fruit of human reflection striving to discern how to live in a way which best respects the kind of persons we are. And the kind of persons we are commits us to facing our responsibilities to the rest of creation as well as to future generations. Moreover, we are becoming much more aware, especially in environmental issues, that what we tend to call 'nature' has already been affected – and, sadly, polluted – by the effects of 'human civilization' over many centuries.

'You are playing God' is an objection often raised when modern technology is applied in some areas of the medical field, for instance in reproductive medicine. The assumption behind this objection seems to be that we should not be interfering with 'nature'. However, a sound theology of creation does not support that assumption. Rather, it reminds us that we are called to exercise responsible stewardship for our world, for ourselves and for future generations. This is our God-given responsibility. God expects us to use our intelligence. In a sense God invites us to 'play God'. It shows little respect for God to use the phrase 'playing God' to mean taking decisions that are likely to harm or even destroy ourselves and our world. That is playing the fool rather than playing God. To me, the phrase 'playing God' reminds us that we are engaged in a God-given task. In a sense, we are continuing God's creative work. That is a tremendous privilege and one we would be abusing if we were not motivated by a determination to do all we could to safeguard and promote the good of humankind, our world and the whole of creation. The wise application of human technology to 'nature' is part of our God-given invitation to 'play God' in the sense of continuing God's creative work in the world. To neglect our responsibility to do this would be to fail to respect who we are as human persons.

Though our bodily givenness is a very important dimension of our nature as human persons, it is not the only one. Our being thinking, evaluating, loving persons is equally part of our nature. Therefore, to be truly human, we need more than an accurate knowledge and understanding of our bodily givenness. We also need to interpret this knowledge and understanding within the broader context of our personal and social relationships according to the best understanding available to us in our contemporary culture. On this point it might be worth repeating a few paragraphs from my book *New Directions in Moral Theology*:

> Philosophically, the natural law does not consist in 'nature' nor even in our knowledge of 'nature'. It consists in our appropriation of this knowledge and our making use of it in trying to discern what kind of personal and social living is most conducive to the safeguarding and promotion of the dignity of human persons . . . This means that the word 'natural' in the term 'natural law' does not refer to natural in contradistinction to artificial. 'Natural' in 'natural law' really means 'reasonable'. In Chapter 3 we considered the eight dimensions of the nature of the human person, integrally and adequately considered. Living as befits a human person means living in a way which takes proper account of all these dimensions of human personhood. Living in this way is living reasonably. It is living in accordance with the natural law.
>
> It is clear from the above that whatever the contraception debate in the Roman Catholic church is about, it should not hinge on the fact that certain methods of contraception are 'artificial'. In itself that has no direct relevance to any natural law discussion. The mere fact that a procedure is 'artificial' does not mean that it is 'unnatural' in terms of the natural law. What is 'artificial' can in fact be more 'natural' in natural law terminology since it can be 'more reasonable'. The 1982 Report *Choices in Childlessness*,

published by the Free Church Federal Council and the British Council of Churches, expressed this point very succinctly:

> ... the popular ethical distinction between the 'natural' and the 'unnatural' is a distinction between what is in keeping with human nature and what is not. It is not a distinction between the natural and the artificial. Since, then, human beings are by nature intelligent and creative, and the adaptation of the environment to their needs is an expression of their intelligence, human artifice, such as that developed in medical technology, is in principle ethically natural. (p. 42)

Furthermore, the notion of 'social construction' links in closely with the social dimension of sin as found in the writings of many theologians today. This is brought out clearly in the following passage from Nicholas Lash, *Believing Three Ways in God* (London, SCM, 1992):

> The world is still unfinished; its history has still some way to go. And there has never been a time, it seems, when all things have been exactly as, according to the Creed, they ought to be. In some sense, then, evil is as old as time. But wickedness is very recent; so is sin – for human beings have not been around for very long. And, even after human malice and stupidity had begun to wreak their havoc, it was not, for many centuries, all that difficult (in principle) to distinguish between 'natural' disasters and the consequences of sin. Now, as the system or structure of the world becomes, increasingly, one complex fact – culturally, politically, technically and economically –, one large *artefact*, one single outcome of human energy and ingenuity, the stain of our malevolence has spread across the surface of the globe. Pollution of the air and seas, deforestation and expansion of the deserts' range, annihilation of innumerable species and exhaustion of non-renewable resources – all these and similar phenomena are caused by human arrogance, short-sightedness and greed. Famine and mass starvation, these days, are no more 'natural' disasters than are deaths caused by the collapse of a building which the landlord neglected to repair. They are the consequences, albeit in some measure unforeseen and unintended, of human action and inaction, of someone's wickedness or sin.
>
> The three concentric circles of non-moral evil, wickedness and sin are rapidly becoming coextensive as the plague of human folly tightens its grip, threatening the planet and the human race with violent, premature, slow death. (pp. 114–15)

Although initially this can sound very depressing, it is, in fact, a helpful reminder to us that theology cannot put creation and redemption into two separate compartments. A natural law approach which focuses solely on the doctrine of creation and ignores the doctrine of redemption will be seriously flawed. That is because the raw material we are handling is not raw at all. It is historically conditioned. It has already been affected by the scenario so vividly portrayed by Lash. While it cannot be denied that we are inheritors of grace, we are also all victims of sin living in a sin-infected world.

Consequently, social construction for the Christian will always remind us that there is a healing task to be undertaken. Salvation necessarily includes the work of 'salvaging'. Unlike God, we are not creating out of nothing. We are wounded healers, handling precious but damaged material. Lash puts this very succinctly when he says that 'the forgiveness of "original" sin is, as we would expect, the finishing of God's creation' (p. 116) or, a little later, 'the world's forgiveness is creation's finishing' (p. 119).

As we shall see in Chapter Four, the approach to 'nature' involved in this kind of theology of creation has profound and very practical implications for our understanding and appreciation of gay and lesbian relationships.

THE CHALLENGE OF GENDER ANALYSIS

Gender analysis uses the notion of social construction to throw light on the process whereby men and women have come to think and behave so differently from each other and how this has affected the way they relate to each other and their respective roles in society. Contrary to popular understanding, gender analysis is not exclusively focused on female gender, as Ursula King brings out very clearly:

> Gender analysis is as much about the construction of male gender roles and identity as it is about female ones, though much less work has been done on the former than the latter. It is about social relations, different sexual orientations, diversity of family patterns, about disruptions and new configurations in gender roles, about the dynamics and flux in cultural symbols, norms and expectations in relation to gender which in turn affect private and public spheres, the world of home and work, the exercise of power and authority. (*Theology and Sexuality*, vol. 3, 1995, p. 116)

Elaine Graham's study, *Making the Difference: Gender, Personhood and Theology* (London, Mowbray, 1995), has made it abundantly clear that gender analysis is a burgeoning science in which there are many different interpretations of the roots of gender differentiation as it currently exists. This reflects the growing conviction that gender differentiation cannot be attributed to any single cause. Graham writes:

> critical analysis of gender consistently challenges notions of a 'unicausal' or reductionist model. Rather, it would appear that the foundations of gender relations and gender identity are complex and multidimensional. (p. 26)

Theologians working in the field of gender analysis would fully accept the contemporary understanding of human sexuality as being a profound dimension of our personhood. We are sexual persons. The meaning of our sexuality is not defined by our reproductive organs. Our sexuality permeates our whole being. In a sense, we are all sexually active from the earliest moments of our life. Our sexuality is about our inner drive to go out of ourselves to others. It is an urge for connectedness. The dynamism of our sexuality plays a major part in our personal and social relationships and even in how we give ourselves to life in general. In her book, *Just Good Friends: Towards a Lesbian and Gay Theology of Relationships* (London, Mowbray, 1995), Elizabeth Stuart borrows from Sally Cline the words of Sister Charles, a vowed celibate, when asked if she would still regard herself as sexual: 'I do not engage in sexual intercourse, but the sexuality I live is like a pulse that goes right through me' (p. 72).

Through understanding sexuality in this broader and much richer sense and using the tools of gender analysis, many theologians have come to the conclusion that our Christian sexual ethics begins from a too limited interpretation of sexuality. It starts from the assumption that our God-given sexuality is essentially bound up with and inseparable from heterosexuality. By heterosexuality is meant the complementarity of men and women as this has been culturally interpreted and embodied in the course of the centuries.

Theologians who query this basic assumption are not challenging the goodness and beauty of marriage, though they, like the rest of us, are fully aware that a marriage can go seriously wrong and can develop into a mutually destructive relationship. Neither are they challenging the value of the family, though here again, like the rest of us, they recognize the enormous shortcomings of families in general and the nuclear family in particular and are aware that today's families come in all shapes and sizes. What they are suggesting is that hetero-sexuality (and still less marriage and the family) might not be the most appropriate starting point for sexual ethics. Perhaps, the fundamental

starting-point should be the human person. And as we have already
seen, in this 'time of AIDS', a person-centred starting-point would
demand a special focus on the dignity of women as human persons.

As we have seen in Chapter One, this starting-point opens our eyes
to the fact that heterosexuality, at least as currently understood and
lived out, does not do full justice to the equal dignity of women and
men. Moreover, this seems to have been the case throughout much
of human history. This is a matter of serious concern, since heterosexuality is seen as one of the most fundamental organizing principles
of society and its various institutions and structures. This is where
gender analysis comes to the rescue. Gender analysis research is
enabling us to see that, though gender is a universal phenomenon,
it is also something which is constructed by human beings themselves.
That is why it is differently nuanced in different societies, cultures and
religions. As a result of her extraordinarily extensive reading in the
field of gender analysis, Elaine Graham argues that we should see
'gender as a form of human practice, natural and cultural' (*Making the
Difference*, p. 155). In other words, gender is not something we are by
nature. It is something human beings have developed in the process of
social living and which as individuals each of us assumes by being part
of this process. Graham quotes Gerda Lerner's account of how this
process might have developed initially:

> The story of civilisation is the story of men and women struggling
> up from necessity, from their helpless dependence on nature, to
> freedom and their partial mastery over nature. In this struggle
> women were longer confined to species-essential activities than
> men and were therefore more vulnerable to being disadvantaged.
> My argument sharply distinguishes between biological necessity,
> to which both men and women submitted and adapted, and
> culturally constructed customs and institutions, which forced
> women into subordinate roles. I have tried to show how it might
> have come to pass that women agreed to a sexual division
> of labour, which would eventually disadvantage them, without
> having been able to foresee the later consequences. (quoted on
> pp. 73–4)

Graham goes on to write:

> Gender is a fundamental form of social organisation. Gender is
> but one manifestation of human social relations; it is not an
> ontological state, nor an intrinsic property of the individual.
> Theories about gender identity, gender regimes and the symbolic
> representations of gender are therefore theories about the

formation of human culture; being a gendered person is about inhabiting a particular culture. Such social relations – and thus gender as a form of social relations – are generated and maintained by human *practice*, symbolic and material . . . Gender is therefore not an innate or ontological category, but the product of human action and social relations, forged by the transformation of the world around us into material and ideological systems. (p. 217)

Thus, human bodies, the practices and conventions of science, religion, language, work, reproduction, families and other social institutions are effectively the agents of gender, in that they are the vehicles by which personal identity is forged within a socially-constructed everyday world. This process is entirely cultural, a constant process of generation and regeneration of social relations. (p. 219)

As we shall see in the next chapter, this approach to gender differentiation, though at odds with the Pope's position on 'ontological complementarity', actually provides a strong ally for the Pope's public call to the whole Church to a 'renewed commitment of fidelity to the Gospel vision' through 'setting women free from every kind of exploitation and domination' (*Letter to Women*, n. 3, in *The Tablet*, 15 July 1985, p. 917). An awareness of the social construction of gender differentiation can make us better equipped to heed the Pope's call since it helps us realize that change and transformation really are possible. And an understanding of the complexity of the whole process will remind us that engagement with it will demand long-term commitment since what is involved is nothing less than a radical transformation of one of the major foundations of civilization as we know it.

The aim of this transformation process is not to eliminate difference between men and women. Nor is it to pursue some kind of holy grail of a pure essence of masculinity and femininity which then becomes the model according to which men and women can fashion their lives. There is no version of masculinity and femininity existing outside of culture. As Graham puts it: 'Whatever human nature may be, it is inaccessible to our understanding beyond the medium of our own culture and agency' (p. 223). The end of the transformation process, therefore, is to re-form gender relations in accordance with the norms of human justice. This involves applying to gender relations a basic principle first formulated by Rosemary Ruether and subsequently strongly affirmed by many other women theologians:

Whatever denies, diminishes, or distorts the full humanity of women is appraised as not redemptive. Theologically speaking, whatever diminishes or denies the full humanity of women must be presumed not to reflect the divine or an authentic relation to the divine, or to reflect the authentic nature of things, or to be the message or work of an authentic redeemer or a community of redemption. (Rosemary Radford Ruether, *Sexism and God-Talk: Towards a Feminist Theology*, London, SCM, 1983, pp. 18–19)

In her final chapter Graham argues paradoxically that, though gender is not founded on 'a God-given order of creation . . . which pre-ordains separate functions for women and men', yet it 'is not merely an incidental aspect of our experience of being human' (p. 223). I would want to express that point theologically by saying that gender is an important dimension of our being human persons which is given to us by God as something which we have to fashion and perfect rather than as a static essence which limits our freedom. To construct gender according to its highest relational possibilities is actually to play our part in the ongoing process of our being created in the image and likeness of God. It is significant that Graham has chosen *Making the Difference* as the title of her book. The word 'making' brings out clearly her key point that gender differentiation is something we make and fashion. A theological version of her title could read *Making the Image of God in Us*. Graham is not unaware of this theological dimension:

The decisive impact of gender as a form of social relations is suggestive of a model of human nature as profoundly relational, requiring the agency of culture to bring our personhood fully into being. This resounds with other perspectives that emphasise such an identity as thoroughly compatible with a Trinitarian model of God. (p. 223)

This is why Christian sexual ethics, at its deepest level, should be about the quality of relationships between sexual persons.

One of the principal ways in which the dignity of the human person is being violated today is through the systematic oppression of women through the all-pervading influence of patriarchy. Therefore, a sexual ethics which starts from the dignity of the human person must, at this point in history, interpret this particularly through the lens of the dignity of women. At present, the playing field is not level in terms of the equality of women and men. That is why we must face the disturbing fact that traditional Christian sexual ethics will almost certainly contain major flaws within it. Otherwise, it could not have been blind to the evil of patriarchy down through the ages. Therefore, it is only to be expected that a transformed Christian sexual ethics, if it is to respect living Christian tradition, will involve a radical reappraisal of certain aspects of what we have considered to be traditional Christian sexual ethics.

3

CHRISTIAN SEXUAL ETHICS AND INJUSTICE AGAINST WOMEN – A CASE OF COLLUSION?

Readers in the developing world might feel that my first chapter had the air of criticizing their culture from a stance of presumed superiority. To counteract that danger, I would like to begin this chapter by showing how Christianity itself grew up in a highly patriarchal cultural milieu and absorbed a patriarchal mind-set into much of its lifestyle, structures and theology. In fact, some even claim that missionary Christianity, far from combating patriarchy in the developing world, actually increased its influence and thereby aggravated the situation still further. Though there are some hopeful signs that things might be changing, it cannot be denied that the legacy of patriarchy is still with us in the Church – and in Western society as a whole.

THE ROOTS OF INJUSTICE AGAINST WOMEN LIE DEEP IN HISTORY

In his book *The Body and Society: Men, Women and Sexual Renunciation in Early Christianity* (London, Faber & Faber, 1988), Peter Brown offers a thoroughly researched and highly acclaimed over-view of the development of attitudes towards sexuality in the early Christian centuries. The picture he paints embodies the kind of complexity one would expect in the development of thought and practice of the newly formed Christian Church as it takes root in different localities and interacts with a variety of philosophical and religious interpretations of the place of sexuality in human life. Naturally, how women fit into this picture is a major feature of his study. Here, too, the picture is complex and far from monochrome. The background which provides the starting-point for his study is very revealing:

In the second century A.D., a young man of the privileged classes of the Roman Empire grew up looking at the world from a position of unchallenged dominance. Women, slaves, and barbarians were unalterably different from him and inferior to him. The most obtrusive polarity of all, that between himself and women, was explained to him in terms of a hierarchy based upon nature itself. (p. 9)

Brown's account of the biological base on which this attitude of male dominance over women was founded is even more startling:

Biologically, the doctrine said, males were those fetuses who had realized their full potential. They had amassed a decisive surplus of 'heat' and fervent 'vital spirit' in the early stages of their coagulation in the womb. The hot ejaculation of male seed proved this: 'For it is the semen, when possessed of vitality, which makes us men, hot, well-braced in limbs, heavy, well-voiced, spirited, strong to think and act.'

Women, by contrast, were failed males. The precious vital heat had not come to them in sufficient quantities in the womb. Their lack of heat made them more soft, more liquid, more clammy-cold, altogether more formless than were men. Periodic menstruation showed that their bodies could not burn up the heavy surpluses that coagulated within them. (pp. 9–10)

Brown comments that these assertions 'had already been made for over half a millennium by this time, and they would continue to be made until this century. They effectively confined women to a lower place than men in an irrefutable, "natural" hierarchy' (p. 10). Moreover, they also helped to explain homophobia in men, since male heat 'unless actively mobilised, might cool, leading even a man to approach the state of a woman' (p. 10). In such a view of the sexual differentiation, for a man to become 'womanish' would be a much-feared form of regression.

This was the thought-world into which early Christianity began to insert itself. While it rejected the male sexual licence which was one possible consequence of such thinking, it took for granted its view of the natural dominance of men over women. Facing the challenge of the Gospel against this background led to a variety of personal and community lifestyles among Christians. Some, like the second-century Gnostic, Valentinus, were so strongly dismissive of women that they portrayed the redemption of women as consisting in their virtually becoming men.

By and large, during the first two centuries the main body of the Church was family based. Naturally, the model of the family here was the patriarchal one accepted in the culture of the time. This would also have been in keeping with the Jewish origins of these Christian communities. It seems to have been only in more radical groups that women had a status on a par with men even if, as with the followers of Valentinus, this was based on their becoming honorary men of a kind. The more settled Christian communities were more likely to follow the rabbinical attitude according to which 'to teach Torah to one's daughter was tantamount to teaching her immorality' (p. 118) and 'it is better to burn Torah than allow a woman to handle it' (p. 145).

The picture changed in the third and fourth centuries, initially through the influence of Origen. His writings, along with those of other bishops and clergy of the period, have left their mark on Christian tradition. With them celibacy began to offer the model for Christian living. At first, this simply meant post-marital celibacy after one's partner had died. However, it quickly turned into a mystique of virginity, understanding it as a single-minded commitment to the Kingdom. Marriage was tolerated as a sin-infected second-best but not a way of life which befitted Church leaders. Paradoxically, in some ways this pro-celibacy attitude helped to promote the equality of women. For instance, the status accorded to post-marriage celibacy gave some wealthy widows the opportunity to gain great influence and play a prominent role in the life of the Christian community. Likewise, the growing attachment to virginity enabled some girls to find an identity for themselves other than the serving role of wife and mother. Nevertheless, within a patriarchal Church, virginity for young women was largely seen from the angle of their not providing a temptation to men. It is no surprise, therefore, to find that when the bishops met at Elvira around 303 a quarter of their decisions were about increased control over the conduct of women in the community.

This concern of the bishops was fully in line with the accepted wisdom that part of the God-given role of men was to control the conduct of women. Women by their nature were called to be naturally submissive to men. This was seen as a basic principle of Church order. This view of women led some to such an extreme as to assert that women were made in the image of men, not of God. That was why the possibility of their being priests was dismissed as 'absurd' by some writers. Evidence of this position is found in the very influential fourth-century commentary on 1 Corinthians by an anonymous Roman priest, commonly referred to as Ambrosiaster:

'Women should keep silence in the church'. In an earlier passage
Paul has ordered that women should be veiled in church. Now he
explains that unless they are quiet and reserved, there is no
purpose in their being veiled. For, if the image of God is man,
and not woman, and if she is subject to man on account of
natural law, how much more in church should she be submissive.
. . . Although woman is one flesh with man, there are two reasons
why she is, nevertheless, ordered to be submissive: first, because
she originated from man; and, secondly, because through her
sin entered the world. (quoted in R. Gryson, *The Ministry of
Women in the Early Church*, Collegeville, MN, The Liturgical Press,
1976, pp. 92–3)

Against such a background it is understandable that the kind of
lifestyle advocated by Eustathius, for a time guide to Basil the Great,
was felt to pose a subversive threat to society and the Church since, as
Brown notes, it 'denied the subjection of women' (*The Body and Society*,
p. 288). The law quickly moved against practices which were seen to
contradict what were considered to be natural symbols of women's
subservience to men:

Women gained their equality by shaving their heads. With the
removal of the 'natural veil' of long hair, so the bishops claimed,
women were encouraged to throw off the sign 'which God gave to
every woman as a reminder of her subjection, thus annulling, as it
were, the ordinance of subjection.' As late as 390, Imperial laws
threatened to depose any bishop who allowed such women into
his church: for 'under the inspiration of their ascetic persuasion
(such women acted) against the laws human and divine'. (Brown,
pp. 288–9)

Within marriage, too, the subordination of women was firmly in place.
For John Chrysostom what mattered most was the right ordering of
hierarchical relationship within the family. This is a far cry from a
relationship based on mutuality and equality between husband and
wife:

The successful running of a Christian household . . . assumed the
dominance of the male within the family, of the husband over his
wife, and of the father over his children. By successfully absorbing
the young wife into his household, the husband would cut her
off from the alluring 'vainglory' of civic life. Gently, but firmly,
she was to be moulded, 'like wax', by her husband. (Brown,
p. 312)

Although prior to his 'conversion', the younger Augustine was for eighteen years faithful to his concubine who bore him a son, Adeodatus (literally, 'the God-given one'), his general attitude to women and their place in marriage and the family seems to imply that women precisely as women are not equal to men. For instance, he states very categorically that he can see no reason other than procreation for God's making women since they are so obviously inferior to men and hence are dispensable in every other respect. His justification for the separate existence of women as distinct from men is seen as a purely functional one:

> If woman has not been made to help man by bearing children, what other kind of help can she give? Not manual labour, since men are better at that than women; nor for company when a man is feeling lonely; another man is much better company and you can have a much more worthwhile conversation with a man than with a woman; not even for the sake of having people who, because naturally submissive to men, are willing to obey orders – when obeying orders is needed, men have shown they can do that just as well as women. So honestly, the only reason I can see why God made women is to bear children. (*De Gen*, ad litt, IX, n. 5)

Moreover, since women provoke the disturbance of sexual arousal in men, Augustine sees them as occasions of sin precisely because of their female sexuality. Hence, even their functionality as channels of procreation is not morally neutral. They cause sexual passion to be aroused in men with the consequent loss of rational control over the body. This is dehumanizing for a man, since it lowers him to the level of brute creation. The power of sin is obviously in operation in such a tragic event and woman is the occasion of this sin. Clearly, this is far from a belief in the full and equal dignity of women. Moreover, Augustine also locates the presence of sin in women not just in their bodily sexuality but also in the disruption of their natural subservience to men. This point is made clearly by the Australian theologian, Kim Power, in her penetrating study on Augustine's attitude to women, *Veiled Desire: Augustine's Writing on Women* (London, Darton, Longman & Todd, 1995):

> When it came to gender relations, Augustine perceived women as inferior and subservient to men, even before the Fall, but he argued that then this subordination would have been a bond of love, a kind of benevolent despotism where men would lead in love and women would love to obey. Since the Fall, this inherent concord is problematic. Spouses may still serve each

other with love, but male domination is mandatory to prevent the increase of corruption and sin. Given his overriding assumptions concerning order, the implication here is that female autonomy, as well as female leadership, has a corrupting effect and would inevitably lead to disorder. (p. 33)

Nevertheless, there is considerable ambiguity, even inconsistency perhaps, in the thought and feelings of Augustine on this topic. At times, he extols the depth of friendship that can exist between men and women, although in marriage he seems to think that this is only achieved through the couple's growing beyond the genital dimension of their relationship. Also, he has a great respect and love for his mother, Monica, and is deeply impressed by the spiritual insights she offers in conversation to himself and his learned male friends.

Many writers have given ample proof that this belief in the inferiority of women and its practical implications for family, Church and society continued down through the centuries right to our own day. It was still alive when I was at seminary in the 1950s. The text-book of moral theology which I studied as part of my preparation for priestly ordination contained the following statement:

> The reason why a woman cannot receive holy orders is because the clerical state demands a certain superiority since it involves ruling the faithful; whereas a woman by her very nature is inferior to man and subject to him. (H. Noldin, *Summa Theologiae Moralis, vol III, De Sacramentis*, Barcelona, Herder, 27th edn, 1951, n. 465)

As will be seen later in the chapter, one of the theological arguments given by the Pope and the Congregation for the Doctrine of the Faith for rejecting the possibility of women being ordained to the priestly ministry is that, 'in the light of what is specific to being male and female', only men can be an 'icon' of Christ. As many theologians, male and female, have pointed out, this line of argument seems to locate the Incarnation in the maleness of Christ rather than in his humanity. Perhaps deep in the Church's unconscious memory, there is still a remnant both of Ambrosiaster's conviction that it is men and not women who really image God and of the fear that right order would be threatened if women were to share equally in ministry and authority in the Church! If that woundedness exists deep in the Church's subconscious memory, the Spirit is surely calling the Church to a healing of memories through women's growing awareness of their full human dignity and through this being acknowledged as one of the 'signs of the times' in our day.

In the next part of this chapter I would like to explore how some recent statements of John Paul II can be seen as signs of hope which could offer a positive contribution towards this healing of memories. However, there is still a long way to go as I hope to show in the final part of this chapter. Responding to the challenge of a 'reconstruction' of gender relationships in the Church needs more than inspiring words. Structural injustice cannot be remedied without radical structural change.

A SIGN OF HOPE: THE 'PRO-WOMEN' TEACHING OF POPE JOHN PAUL II

In a number of statements in 1995 in connection with the United Nations' 4th World Conference on Women in Beijing, Pope John Paul II committed himself to a public recognition of the 'pro-women' moral imperative of our age. For instance, in his message of 26 May 1995 to the UN Conference presented to its Secretary General, Mrs Gertrude Mongella (text in *Briefing*, 17 August 1995, pp. 16–18), he states:

> Solutions to the issues and problems raised at the conference, if they are to be honest and permanent, cannot but be based on *the recognition of the inherent, inalienable dignity of women,* and the importance of women's presence and participation in all aspects of social life. (n. 2, italics as in text)

The Pope also acknowledges that for the full dignity of women to be given true recognition at a practical level, structural changes will need to be made within society:

> Profound changes are needed in the attitudes and organisation of society in order to facilitate the participation of women in public life, while at the same time providing for the special obligations of women and men with regard to their families. In some cases changes have also to be made to render it possible for women to have access to property and to the management of their assets. (n. 5)

This leads the Pope to insist that 'greater efforts are needed to eliminate discrimination against women in areas that include education, health care and employment' (n. 6). He also denounces '*the terrible exploitation of women and girls* which exists in every part of the world' (n. 7) and singles out for special mention the sexual exploitation of women. A striking passage in the Pope's message states that the full recognition of the equal dignity of women and men will not be properly respected unless its financial implications are faced. He even suggests that a deregulated free-market economy is more likely to exploit women rather than to promote their true equality:

> Women's greater presence in the work force, in public life, and generally in the decision-making processes guiding society, on an equal basis with men, will continue to be problematic as long as the costs continue to burden the private sector ... In the perspective of uncontrolled free-market policies there is little hope that women will be able to overcome the obstacles on their path. (n. 8)

What is particularly significant for the issues under consideration in this chapter is the Pope's advertence to 'social and cultural conditioning' which, he says, 'does not permit women to become aware of their own dignity, with drastic consequences for the proper balance of society and with continuing pain and despair on the part of so many women' (n. 8). The Pope's point about social conditioning denying women access to the appreciation of their own dignity is taken up by Professor Mary Ann Glendon, Head of the Holy See's Delegation, in her opening address at Beijing (text in *Briefing*, 19 October 1995, pp. 16–19). She applauds the draft *Platform of Action* for its commitment 'to free women at last from the unfair burdens of cultural conditioning that have so often prevented them even from becoming conscious of their own dignity' (n. 1).

Professor Glendon's point about the enormous harm suffered by women as a result of cultural conditioning is made even more forcefully in the Pope's *Letter to Women* issued on the 29 June 1995 (text in *The Tablet*, 15 July 1995, pp. 917–19). There he acknowledges that the Church has played a part in this 'anti-woman' cultural conditioning and actually offers a public apology for it:

> Unfortunately, we are heirs to a history which has conditioned us to a remarkable extent. In every time and place, this conditioning has been an obstacle to the progress of women. Women's dignity has often been unacknowledged and their prerogatives misrepresented; they have often been relegated to the margins of society and even reduced to servitude. This has prevented women from truly being themselves and it has resulted in a spiritual impoverishment of humanity. Certainly it is no easy task to assign the blame for this, considering the many kinds of cultural conditioning which down the centuries have shaped ways of thinking and acting. And if objective blame, especially

in particular historical contexts, has belonged to not just a few members of the Church, for this I am truly sorry. May this regret be transformed, on the part of the whole Church, into a renewed commitment of fidelity to the Gospel vision. (n. 3)

After a deeply felt and obviously well-meant but slightly patronizing series of 'thank you's to women in various walks of life, the remainder of the first half of the letter constitutes a very powerful statement of the full and equal dignity of women and an impassioned denunciation of the ways in which women's dignity continues to be violated today. A few quotations should amply demonstrate the strong 'pro-women' character of this section of the letter:

> There is an urgent need to achieve real equality in every area: equal pay for equal work, protection for working mothers, fairness in career advancements, equality of spouses with regard to family rights and the recognition of everything that is part of the rights and duties of citizens in a democratic state. This is a matter of justice but also of necessity. (n. 4)
>
> How can we not mention the long and degrading history, albeit often an 'underground' history, of violence against women in the area of sexuality? At the threshold of the third millennium we cannot remain indifferent and resigned before this phenomenon. The time has come to condemn vigorously the types of sexual violence which frequently have women for their object and to pass laws which effectively defend them from such violence. Nor can we fail, in the name of respect due to the human person, to condemn the widespread hedonistic and commercial culture which encourages the systematic exploitation of sexuality and corrupts even very young girls into letting their bodies be used for profit. (n. 5)

Similar points are made by Professor Glendon in her Beijing opening address:

> Women must be guaranteed measures of economic and social security which reflect their equal dignity, their equal rights to ownership of property and access to credit and resources. The effective contribution of women's work to economic security and social well-being is often greater than that of men. (*Briefing*, p. 17)
>
> The majority of those who today live in abject poverty are women and children. Efforts must be strengthened to eliminate all those cultural and legal obstacles which impair the economic

security of women . . . No part of the world is without its scandal of poverty which strikes women most . . . The 'feminisation of poverty' must be of concern to all women. Its social, political and economic roots must be addressed. (p. 18)

Concerned women must take the lead in the fight against societal practices which facilitate the irresponsibility of men while stigmatising women, and against a vast industry that extracts its profits from the very bodies of women, while at the same time purporting to be their liberators . . . More must be done to eliminate the practice of female genital mutilation. (p. 19)

Noting the attitude of Jesus Christ himself who 'transcended the norms of his own culture and treated women with openness, respect, acceptance and tenderness', the Pope puts a challenging question before the whole Church at the end of the second millennium: 'How much of his message has been heard and acted upon?' By referring to this moment in history, 'at the end of this millennium', the Pope seems to be making his own the conviction of Paul VI that one of the major 'signs of the times' for our day is the growing consciousness among women of their full and equal dignity as human persons and the movement among them to break free from attitudes, beliefs and practices which explicitly or implicitly contradict this dignity. The Pope seems to be saying that if we want to hear the message of Christ for our day we must listen respectfully to what these inspired women are saying and recognize the action of God's Spirit at work in their movement for liberation.

There is a growing conviction among many Christians, including many theologians, that 'the time of AIDS' is a *kairos* time, a defining moment. This challenging insight seems to have originated with the Irish theologian, Enda McDonagh, a member of the Caritas Internationalis AIDS Task Force. He has explored its implications in numerous talks across the world and in various articles he has written (cf. 'Theology in a time of AIDS', in *Irish Theological Quarterly*, 1994, pp. 81–99 and reprinted in his *Faith in Fragments*, Maynooth Bicentenary Series, Dublin, Columba Press, 1996, chap. 11). Understanding the present as a *kairos* moment in a theological sense means seeing it as a time in which we are being offered the opportunity to play our part in one of God's mighty wonders. In the context of what the Pope has said, I would suggest that there is a convergence of two impulses of the Spirit taking place here. We are living in 'a time of AIDS' and we are also living in 'a time of women'. Though each of these *kairos* moments may contain its own specific challenge and opportunity, nevertheless, there is a considerable overlap between them.

This seems to be particularly true in the realm of Christian sexual ethics. I believe that we cannot really hear the challenge to sexual ethics found in 'the time of AIDS' unless there is the full participation of women in this interpretative listening process. It is as though the experience-based theological reflection of women is fashioning a clearer lens enabling the Church to see what needs to be done. In other words, if we were not living in an age in which God's Spirit is speaking in new ways through the voices of women interpreting their own experience, the Church might not be able to interpret accurately what God's Spirit is saying in 'the time of AIDS'. To be more specific, in so far as theology, including moral theology, is still dominated by men and moral teaching is formulated and articulated almost exclusively by men, male theologians and the men invested with episcopal teaching authority must listen to the voices of women inter-preting their own experience. Moreover, women must have a full and equal role in the deliberations arising out of this process. Today it is the critical analysis of women rather than the solutions of men which must be listened to. This is not an abdication of theological integrity or teaching authority. It is simply responding to a movement of God's Spirit enabling the Church to be more truly itself through empowering women and men equally to reflect more truly in their lives the relational God in whose image we are all created.

THE POPE AND GENDER: HOW COMPLIMENTARY TO WOMEN IS ONTOLOGICAL COMPLEMENTARITY?

The Pope's *Letter to Women* provoked a variety of reactions among women. A selection of these are found in *The Tablet*, 15 July 1995, pp. 920–1. Some, like Pat Jones, were encouraged by the letter's general tone, its acknowledgement of the harm done to women by social conditioning, its willingness to apologize for the Church's part in this and the sign it gives that 'the Church is reaching for a new language and a deeper dialogue about men and women, and our social and personal relationships'. Others, like Pia Buxton, were more muted in their welcome, pointing out the pain and confusion caused by the fact that 'the Church's teaching may be experienced as contradictory and at variance with its practice'.

Understandably, many women were saddened, some even angered, by the Pope's insistence once again on the notion of 'ontological complementarity' to explain the gender differentiation between men and women. Clearly, much of the Pope's letter could only have been written as a result of his careful listening to the voices of women articulating their experiences of oppression. Hence, women theologians found it difficult to understand how, on this particular point, he seemed unable to hear what they were saying in the light of their own experience and that of their sisters.

By incorporating the notion of 'ontological complementarity' into his theology, the Pope is choosing one particular view among many in the area of gender analysis. Moreover, it is a view which is rejected by the majority of women theologians since it does not correspond to their own experience and that of most other women. The theory of 'ontological complementarity' maintains that the distinction between men and women has been so designed by God that they complement each other, not just in their genital sexual faculties but also in their minds and hearts and in the particular qualities and skills they bring to life, and specifically to family life. In other words, it necessarily predisposes men and women to mutually complementary roles within marriage and family life in such a way that this role-predisposition is an intrinsic part of their personal identity and will always influence their behaviour, even if they never actually undertake this role. In practice, this would mean that the thinking and behaviour of women will be strongly coloured by their predisposition to motherhood. As we have already seen, Christian tradition has interpreted the roles of father and mother through a patriarchal-coloured lens.

Kim Power makes this point very powerfully in her above-mentioned study of Augustine:

> In recent decades, religious attitudes to women, encoded in canonical texts, have been made more conscious and overt in the debates over the liturgical participation and ordination of women. From these it has become clear that although the Catechisms might proclaim that all human beings are made in the image and likeness of God, this is not necessarily interpreted as applying to men and women in the same way . . .

> The ontological inferiority of women found in the ancient texts has been supplanted by the argument from complementarity. Woman is now equal but different, and the difference determines her destiny and her subordination . . .

Both ancient and modern writings appeal to a biological determinism to legitimate the structures of power in heterosexual social relations. In both, the explanation of woman's nature is totally male-defined, that is, androcentric. Androcentrism is any mode of thinking, understanding or expression which is formed almost exclusively by male experience and understanding and which identifies male experience with 'human' experience. (*Veiled Desire*, p. 4)

The 'ontological complementarity' interpretation highlights certain specific aspects of gender difference, as popularly envisaged by many people today, and endows these different characteristics with a timeless and unchanging character. They are presented as constituting the 'essence' of being a man or a woman. As we have already noted, the trouble with this position is that it overlooks the fact that our gender difference as we experience it today is the product of the process of social construction down through the ages. This makes it impossible for us to isolate out any particular factors as pertaining to the timeless essence of being a man or a woman. Ultimately, the 'ontological complementarity' position is oppressive and deterministic since it implies that we cannot examine critically whether the gender roles we receive as given today are not, in fact, the end-product of an ongoing process of social construction and therefore open to further trans-formation in the light of what is in keeping with the dignity of human persons.

Women theologians do not deny the obvious fact that men and women are different. However, they are saying that the 'ontological complementarity' view put forward by the Pope and shared uncritically by many Christians is not a true interpretation of reality since it over-simplifies the complexity of the phenomenon of gender differentiation. For most women theologians the Pope's position is an instance of the kind of 'unicausal' reductionist approach criticized by Elaine Graham for failing to do justice to the multidimensional factors at play (cf. *supra*, p. 35). Moreover, it seems to imply that the very heart of being a woman lies in her being complementary to man. This comes perilously close to a definition based on deficiency. It seems to suggest that to be a woman is to be someone designed to complement men and needing the complementarity of men for completion. Of course, the same objection can be raised about defining men in this way. Women theologians are not denying that complementarity is an aspect of being a woman or a man but they are claiming that it does not get to the heart of what it means to be a woman – or a man, for that matter.

Moreover, in practice the ontological complementarity approach unconsciously tends to collude in the kind of oppression the Pope has been denouncing so vehemently. In this way, it can constitute an obstacle to the genuine liberation of women which the Pope sees as a Gospel imperative for our day.

Many women also reacted against the way the Pope used the notion of 'ontological complementarity' to rule out the ordination of women to the ministerial priesthood. He argued that their exclusion was based on 'the "iconic" complementarity of male and female roles' (*Letter to Women*, n. 11). Although the main thrust of his argument is that Christ only ordained men and the Church must follow his example, nevertheless, he seems to suggest that, in so doing, Christ and his Church are conforming to the natural or ontological order of 'what is specific to being male and female'. For instance, he teaches that 'Christ ... entrusted only to men the task of being an "icon" of his countenance as "shepherd" and "bridegroom" of the Church through the exercise of the ministerial priesthood'. However, he prepares the ground for this assertion by stating that 'the presence of a certain diversity of roles is in no way prejudicial to women, provided that this diversity is not the result of an arbitrary imposition, but is rather an expression of what is specific to being male and female' (n. 11). Hence, there seems some ambiguity in the Pope's claim that the ineligibility of women for the priesthood is based on 'Christ's free and sovereign choice'.

Furthermore, there is a certain inconsistency in the Pope's stance on 'ontological complementarity'. He rightly observes that 'we are heirs to a history which has conditioned us to a remarkable extent' and that 'in every time and place, this conditioning has been an obstacle to the progress of women'. However, if that is true, it follows that no element in gender differentiation as currently operating can be regarded as immune from this historical conditioning. That means that if we are to subject this historical conditioning to critical appraisal, we will need to introduce some kind of external bench-mark to act as our criterion of evaluation. That is precisely what the Pope does when he appeals to 'respect due to the human person' in order to criticize our contemporary culture for its exploitation of women. However, the inconsistency in his position, as noted by women theologians, is that he fails to apply that same criterion to the specific factors of gender differentiation which he isolates out as constituting the essence of being a woman. In real life, women actually experience the effects of this 'ontological complementarity' approach as oppressive and contradictory to their dignity as human persons. That is why they would challenge the Pope with his own words:

> one can also appreciate that the presence of a certain diversity of roles is in no way prejudicial to women, provided that this diversity is not the result of an arbitrary imposition, but is rather an expression of what is specific to being male and female. (*Letter to Women*, n. 11, in *The Tablet*, 15 July 1995, p. 919)

Most women theologians claim that the teaching of the Pope on the complementary roles which he sees as specific to men and women is, in their personal experience as women, 'prejudicial to women'. They regard it as 'an arbitrary imposition'. And, in the case of the exclusion of women from the ministerial priesthood, this 'arbitrary imposition' is even given the ultimate seal of divine approval by suggesting that it is grounded in 'Christ's free and sovereign choice'.

A discussion of the ordination of women might seem out of place in a book exploring new directions in sexual ethics in the light of the AIDS pandemic. However, I hope the above analysis shows that the exclusion of women from the priesthood seems to be linked to the kind of mind-set which we saw in Chapter One to be at odds with the full and equal dignity of women and, as such, undergirding cultural attitudes and practices which leave women very exposed to HIV infection.

THE EXPERIENCE OF WOMEN

Since sexual ethics is about being true to who we are as sexual persons, this means that at certain moments in history its focus will be much more on liberation from sexually oppressive structures and behaviour than on formulating universal norms. The 'time of AIDS' and the 'time of women' together constitute such a moment. That is why I am arguing that the focus of a Christian sexual ethic for today will be mainly on liberating women – and men – from the oppressive and dehumanizing influence of everything that goes to make up patriarchy. As we have seen, one of those things is heterosexuality, understood in the sense of 'ontological complementarity'. Patriarchy needs heterosexuality as one of its building blocks. The sexes need to be clearly distinct if the superiority of men over women is to operate effectively.

The way this critical analysis seems to have come about among some women is through reflecting upon their experience of sexual relationships. They have come to realize that what most women have been looking for has been a deep and enduring personal relationship, lived out in a spirit of mutuality and equality. What many women have, in fact, experienced has been a relationship based on power, exploitation and manipulation. Very often they have felt they have been 'used', either for pleasure or for procreation. Their experience of marriage has frequently been that of being 'owned' by their husband. As we have seen, this notion has a long history and is still very much alive, though more blatant in some cultures than in others.

Reflecting on their own experience has led many women to become aware that where they most fully experience equality and mutuality in a relationship is with one or other of their women friends. Their best friend is actually another woman. Elizabeth Stuart notes that 'in the 1987 Hite Report on *Women and Love*, a staggering 87 per cent of married women and 95 per cent of single women claimed that they had their deepest emotional relationship with a woman friend' (*Just Good Friends*, p. 97). For the most part, though these women have a deep and affectionate love for each other, they do not feel any desire to give this love any kind of genital expression. Nevertheless, reflecting on this experience has raised serious questions for them in the field of sexual ethics. Why do they enjoy an equal and mutual relationship with a woman friend when they do not relate to their husbands in the same way? Is this saying something about the male–female sexual (i.e. heterosexual) relationship? Are the intrinsic dynamics of that relationship necessarily bound up with notions of domination and conquest on the one hand, and submission and manipulation on the other?

Women theologians refuse to answer 'Yes' to this last question. Even if this is how many heterosexual relationships operate, they would claim that this need not necessarily be the case. This oppressive model of heterosexuality is a social construction and, as such, it is open to reconstruction. Such liberating reconstruction is part of the practical agenda arising from Christian feminist theology. Moreover, these women theologians would refuse to answer 'Yes' to that same question on theological grounds as well. As Christians we believe we are relational persons created in the image of a relational God. Hence, they would argue that our model for relationship is essentially one of mutuality and interdependence between persons who are equal, though distinct and unique.

Although the way into this Christian feminist critique has been

through rejecting the sexual oppression of women in all its ramifica-
tions, it eventually arrives at a point where it is challenging Christian
sexual ethics to be truer to its real theological foundations.
Christian sexual ethics has been too uncritical in its acceptance of
heterosexuality as its basic starting-point. It has too readily assumed
that the only truly human sexual relationship is that between a man
and a woman. Any sexual relationship deviating from that norm is a
deviant relationship, with 'deviant' here meaning ethically deviant in
the sense of contradicting what it means to be truly human and not
merely socially deviant in the sense of being a minority behaviour.
What many women theologians are suggesting is that we need to
explore whether, theologically, what might be morally deviant is
heterosexuality itself, at least in some of the ways it is currently lived
out and embodied in our different cultures and institutions. Clearly,
this issue is also one of major concern to gay theologians too. However,
it would only confuse the discussion if I introduced their experience-
based reflections at this juncture. The following chapter will examine
their thinking in more detail.

This long discussion of heterosexuality as a social construct might
seem light-years removed from the plight of many of the women
affected by HIV/AIDS mentioned in the first part of this essay.
However, a little reflection will show that they are intimately
connected.

In Chapter One we saw how it is the inferior status of these women
which has left them prey to HIV/AIDS. This inferior status is not
due to any personal deficiency in them as individuals. It is due to the
fact that they are women and that, in their cultures, women are
regarded as second-class citizens. They are subject to sexual and
economic subordination. This is patriarchy in action. The precise form
this sexual and economic subordination takes needs to be examined
critically in each culture. How precisely women are viewed as different
from men may well vary from culture to culture, but the common
thread linking them all seems to be that what makes women different
also makes them inferior. Hence, they are subordinate to men and
subject to them. This has practical implications in those areas of life
where women and men come into contact with each other – marriage,
family, school, work-place, medicine, politics and, of course, religion.
I say 'and, of course, religion' because religion normally seems to
play an important role in legitimating this system of gender differentiation. In some way or other religion tends to interpret it as 'divinely
ordained'. Alison Webster makes a thought-provoking observation

in this connection: 'When a particular ideal is labelled "God-given" the immediate effect is to discourage exploration of its origin and rationale. We are diverted from asking crucial questions about whose interests are served by it' (*Found Wanting: Women, Christianity and Sexuality*, London, Cassell, 1995, p. 42).

The theory of social construction in general, but particularly its application to gender differentiation, can provide the key to open the prison door of a culture which is experienced by women as oppressive. It enables women to see their oppression as the result of history rather than of destiny. And since history is formed by human hands, it can also be re-formed by human hands.

The seed of hope sown by this transition from destiny to social construction can be brought to life by the insight that liberating engagement with the process of social construction actually is a response to the will of God as made known to us today. In other words, what is 'divinely ordained' is not something static and unalterable, namely, heterosexuality in the oppressive ways in which it is currently experienced by many women. Rather, what is 'divinely ordained' is the dynamic and liberating mission of reconstructing gender relations in a way which is more in keeping with the human dignity of every human person. Moreover, increasingly it is becoming appreciated that patriarchy in its various guises is dehumanizing for men as well as for women. Since we are relational beings through and through, men's relationship with women will not be the enriching experience it can be if it is distorted by false notions of male superiority and female inferiority or by denying each other the freedom to break out of socially constructed gender roles. Hence, the transformative practice of liberating cultures from their oppressive patriarchal dimension is as much the concern of men as it is of women. Professor Mary Ann Glendon, Head of the Holy See's Delegation to the 1995 Beijing UN Conference on Women, began her opening address by stressing her delegation's belief that the outcome of such a transformation of society will be of enormous benefit to all:

> The historical oppression of women has deprived the human race of untold resources. Recognition of the equality in dignity and fundamental rights of women and men, and guaranteeing access by all women to the full exercise of those rights will have far-reaching consequences and will liberate enormous reserves of intelligence and energy sorely needed in a world that is groaning for peace and justice. (n. 1, in *Briefing*, 19 October 1995, p. 16)

She returns to the same point at the end of her address when she says that 'the freer women are to share their gifts with society, and to assume leadership in society, the better are the prospects for the entire human community to progress in wisdom, justice and dignified living' (n. 4, *Briefing*, p. 19).

COLLUSION WITH INJUSTICE AGAINST WOMEN?

One of the points I have been arguing in this chapter is that sexual ethics is about more than specific norms for sexual behaviour. Much more fundamentally it is about dismantling the cultural conditioning which, in the words of John Paul II, 'has prevented women from truly being themselves and has resulted in a spiritual impoverishment of humanity' (*Letter to Women*, n. 3). I believe the Pope gives very high priority to this task which he sees as being bound up with 'fidelity to the Gospel vision' (loc. cit.). In other words, for him this is an essential part of the Good News of the Gospel.

As we have already seen, the Pope is wedded to the notion of 'ontological complementarity'. In no way does he see this as violating the equal dignity of women. I believe that, if he did, he would change his view immediately. However, at present, he seems unable to hear women theologians telling him that, in practice, the kind of 'ontological complementarity' he espouses is experienced by them as oppressive and fails to do justice to their true dignity as human persons. Though he does not see it this way at present, it might be part of that cultural conditioning for which the Pope, in his *Letter to Women*, is prepared, on behalf of the Church, to accept 'objective blame' and say 'I am truly sorry'.

The Pope's version of 'ontological complementarity' differs somewhat from that held in the early Church and in subsequent centuries. However, it still needs to be looked at with a critical eye. An understanding of the process of social construction helps us appreciate that gender differentiation is simply part of a wider and much more complex pattern of social relationships. This comes out even in the way the structures of the Church operate. In practice, maintaining the inadmissibility of women to the ministerial priesthood has had the result that, for the most part, women have been marginalized when it comes to important levels of decision-making in the Church. This has been true at all levels of the Church's life. In practice, the inadmissibility of women to ordination involves also, for the most part, the inadmissibility of women to the exercise of power and leadership in the Church.

It would seem, therefore, that on this issue, at least, the Church in its own internal life and structures needs to be counter-cultural. Both the Pope and Professor Mary Ann Glendon have strongly challenged the nations of the world to set in motion radical changes to combat injustice against women. Sadly, with only minimal re-wording, those same challenges could legitimately be made to the Church with regard to its own internal life and structures. For instance, in his message to Mrs Mongella for the Beijing conference the Pope spoke of 'the importance of women's presence and participation in all aspects of social life' (n. 2, cf. *Briefing*, 17 August 1995, p. 16) and shared his belief that 'when women are able fully to share their gifts with the whole community, the very way in which society understands and organises itself is improved' (n. 5, *Briefing*, p. 17). Earlier, in his *Letter to Women*, he had stressed the 'urgent need (for women) to achieve equality in every area' (n. 4). Moreover, in her opening address at Beijing, Professor Glendon voiced the Holy See's support for 'the right of women to effectively enjoy equal opportunities and conditions with men in the workplace as well as in the decision-making structures of society, especially as they affect women themselves' (n. 2).

All these statements are immensely important and constitute a radical challenge to society to transform its oppressive approach to gender differentiation. That is all the more reason why these same statements should also be heard as a radical challenge to the Church itself to undertake a similar reform within its own life and structures.

One hopeful sign that this is beginning to be recognized among men in the Church can be seen in the 14th Decree, 'Jesuits and the situation of women in Church and civil society', of the 34th Congregation of the Jesuits held in Rome, January–March, 1995. After analysing the situation, this decree states:

> (9) We Jesuits first ask God for the grace of conversion. We have been part of a civil and ecclesial tradition that has offended against women. And, like many men, we have a tendency to convince ourselves that there is no problem. However unwittingly, we have often contributed to a form of clericalism which has reinforced male domination with an ostensibly divine sanction. By making this declaration we wish to react personally and collectively, and do what we can to change this regrettable situation. (n. 369)

A little later it offers some specific ways forward:

(12) In the first place, we invite all Jesuits to listen carefully and courageously to the experience of women. Many women feel that men simply do not listen to them. There is no substitute for such listening. More than anything else it will bring about change. Unless we listen, any action we may take in this area, no matter how well intentioned, is likely to bypass the real concerns of women and to confirm male condescension and reinforce male dominance. Listening, in a spirit of partnership and equality, is the most practical response we can make and is the foundation for our mutual partnership to reform unjust structures.

(13) Second, we invite all Jesuits, as individuals and through their institutions, to align themselves in solidarity with women. The practical ways of doing this will vary from place to place and from culture to culture, but many examples come readily to mind:

1. explicit teaching of the essential equality of women and men in Jesuit ministries, especially in schools, colleges and universities;
2. support for liberation movements which oppose the exploitation of women and encourage their entry into political and social life;
3. specific attention to the phenomenon of violence against women;
4. appropriate presence of women in Jesuit ministries and institutions, not excluding the ministry of formation;
5. genuine involvement of women in consultation and decision-making in our Jesuit ministries;
6. respectful cooperation with our female colleagues in shared projects;
7. use of appropriately inclusive language in speech and official documents;
8. promotion of the education of women and, in particular, the elimination of all forms of illegitimate discrimination between boys and girls in the education process.

(*Documents of the 34th General Congregation of the Society of Jesus*, Saint Louis, Institute of Jesuit Sources, 1995, pp. 174–6)

I cannot help thinking that the log-jam in the Church is located in its stance on 'ontological complementarity' and in the powerful way this is symbolized in its teaching on the inadmissibility of women for priestly ordination. There may or may not be many women in the Church who believe they are called to this form of ministry. That is beside the point for our present discussion. The real point is that, in this 'time of women', the inadmissibility of women to the ministerial priesthood should only be presented as belonging to the deposit of faith if it can be shown to be an integral and essential element of the

Gospel which has consistently been heard and experienced as 'good news' by women down through the ages. I believe that the opposite has been the case. Far from being an integral element of the 'good news' it seems more like part of that cultural conditioning down the centuries which the Pope refers to as 'an obstacle to the progress of women'.

Despite recent set-backs to positive movement here, I believe that the Church as a whole, and Pope John Paul II in particular, are moving in a forward direction. A few weeks before the Beijing Conference, the Pope made an impassioned appeal to the whole Church to enhance the role of women in its own internal life:

> Today I appeal to the whole Church community to be willing to foster *feminine participation* in every way in its internal life . . .
>
> The 1987 Synod on the laity expressed precisely this need and asked that 'without discrimination women should be participants in the life of the Church and also in consultation and the process of coming to decisions'. (*Propositio* 47; cf. *Christifideles laici*, n. 51)
>
> To a large extent, it is a question of making full use of the *ample* room for a lay and feminine presence recognised by the Church's law. I am thinking, for example of theological teaching, the forms of liturgical ministry permitted, including service at the altar, pastoral and administrative councils, Diocesan Synods and Particular Councils, various ecclesial institutions, curias, and ecclesiastical tribunals, many pastoral activities, including the new forms of participation in the care of parishes when there is a shortage of clergy, except for those tasks that belong properly to the priest. (*L'Osservatore Romano*, English edition, 6 September 1995, p. 1)

It was this address of the Pope that prompted the editor of the *National Catholic Reporter* to suggest some concrete steps which the Pope himself could take to promote this process. In addition to appointing women to head some of Vatican Curia congregations, the editor suggests that the Pope might name some women members to the College of Cardinals, a suggestion also made by Maureen MacGlashan, the British Ambassador to the Holy See (cf. Annabel Miller, 'Women in the Vatican', in *The Tablet*, 29 March/2 April 1997, pp. 428–30 at p. 430). The *National Catholic Reporter* editor points out that the only official function of the college is to elect the next pope and argues that 'no longer should Catholic women be voiceless in the choice of the person to lead their church'. Such a step would pose no theological problem and would only require a minor change in some recent canons in Church law:

> Making a woman a cardinal at a time when women cannot be priests would seem to be an impossibility. But not so. There is precedent for lay cardinals, although they have all been men. Lay cardinals were common during the Renaissance. The last cardinal who was not a priest at the time of his appointment was Giacomo Antonelli, a church deacon and secretary of state to Pope Pius IX. He died in 1876. (*National Catholic Reporter*, 15 September 1995, p. 24)

A further comment by the same editor pin-points the relevance of this suggestion to the theme of this book: 'No modern pope has made issues of sexual morality and gender more central to church orthodoxy. This is all the more reason for Catholic women to be involved in decisions related to these and other matters.'

Not so long ago, in order to stand up for their basic social, economic and political rights women had to disregard those who told them that what they were doing was a sin. Such women have received great praise from the Pope in his *Letter to Women*:

> I cannot fail to express my admiration for those women of good will who have devoted their lives to defending the dignity of womanhood by fighting for their basic social, economic and political rights, demonstrating courageous initiative at a time when this was considered extremely inappropriate, the sign of a lack of feminity, a manifestation of exhibitionism, and even a sin. (n. 6, in *The Tablet*, 15 July 1995, p. 918)

The Pope here implies that these women were right to disregard those who told them that what they were doing was sinful. Perhaps women today who disregard the reply of the Congregation for the Doctrine of the Faith and continue believing in and working for the ordination of women will be similarly praised by some future Pope!

More than 40,000 women from all over the world converged on Beijing for the 1995 UN 4th World Conference on Women. Its *Platform for Action* statement constitutes a very comprehensive check-list of the kind of action that needs to be taken to ensure that the full equality of women becomes a reality at every level of society in our world. As such, it offers some extremely important suggestions for the agenda of building God's Kingdom in our world today (cf. Joan Chittister, *Beyond Beijing: The Next Step for Women*, Kansas City, Sheed & Ward, 1996). Consequently, if Christian Churches are to be attentive to God's word as it is spoken to us today, they must study this Beijing statement very carefully. Although its moral imperatives are directed specifically to governments, they also have important implications for Christian Churches and their members. We have already seen that, in the light of the global situation with regard to the status of women and the tragedy and injustice resulting from this with regard to HIV/AIDS, a guiding principle for Christian sexual ethics at this moment in time should be that the Church must be pro-women before it is pro-marriage. Maybe the Beijing statement can help to put some flesh and blood on that principle. For instance, perhaps no Christian Church should issue any further statement about marriage or sexual ethics until it has first produced a down-to-earth practical statement committing itself to what John Paul II describes as 'setting women free from every kind of exploitation and domination' and explicitly considering the implications of the Beijing *Platform for Action* for its own life. Obviously, such a statement would lack all credibility if women members of the Church were not allowed to collaborate in a major way in its production.

4

SEXUAL ETHICS – DENYING THE GOOD
NEWS TO GAY MEN AND LESBIAN WOMEN?

THE LINK BETWEEN PATRIARCHY AND
HOMOPHOBIA

Tragically, many gay men, especially in the United States, have been infected with HIV and the death toll among the gay community has been devastating. In the light of this, it might seem natural to have a chapter on homosexuality in a book of essays responding to the HIV/AIDS pandemic. However, that explanation could give the impression that this chapter has nothing in common with the gender issues about women which we explored in the previous chapter. That is far from true.

A gay relationship is commonly perceived in terms of one partner taking on the subordinate role of a woman. Men see that as a form of betrayal. It introduces a Trojan Horse into the stronghold of patriarchy. It breaks what is seen to be the natural order of things since it involves one male partner adopting the subordinate role of a woman and the other partner being willing to collude in this betrayal of male identity. Gareth Moore believes that the roots of opposition to male homosexual behaviour in the Bible go back to this socially constructed patriarchal foundation (cf. *The Body in Context: Sex and Catholicism*, London, SCM, 1992, pp. 38–42). He even suggests that this is why the Bible shows so little interest in lesbians. The link between patriarchy and homophobia is also pointed out by William D. Lindsey:

> the manifold forms of violence our society practices against gay people presuppose that nexus of social structures and attitudes feminist thinkers identify as patriarchy. A primary task of theologians concerned to seek justice for gay people is clearly to show what hides within much anti-gay rhetoric: to show that such

rhetoric is often not really about sexuality so much as it is about maintaining patriarchy . . . Christian moral theologians cannot continue to talk about the morality of homosexuality as if something more is not present in all that church and society say about homosexuality . . . And that something more is not merely homophobia: it is also misogyny, a haughty disdain for *anything* perceived by patriarchy as feminine . . . ('The AIDS crisis and the Church: a time to heal', in *Theology and Sexuality*, no. 2, March 1995, p. 28)

THE DISSIMILARITY OF LESBIAN AND GAY EXPERIENCE

Elizabeth Stuart pushes this line of thought still further. After noting that 'homophobia has its roots in the patriarchal fear of female sexuality' (*Just Good Friends*, p. 23), she points out that some women choose to identify themselves as lesbian precisely as a rejection of the whole patriarchal portfolio:

A lesbian, by refusing to play the role assigned to women in a patriarchal context, exposes the patriarchal understanding of women to be a social construct, and thereby subverts it. And so we can begin to understand why some women who would not be defined as 'lesbian' by a society which thinks of lesbian as 'a homosexual woman', and regards homosexuality as 'feeling or involving sexual attraction only to persons of the same sex', would choose to identify as lesbian, or steadfastly refuse the label 'heterosexual', as a personal political statement. (*Just Good Friends*, p. 71; cf. also Rosemary Ruether in Jeannine Gramick ed., *Homosexuality in the Priesthood and the Religious Life*, New York, Crossroad, 1989, p. 28)

The experience of lesbian women, therefore, may be very different from that of gay men. As Stuart points out, gay men are still men and, to that extent, continue to enjoy many of the 'privileges' of patriarchy:

No one can doubt that lesbians and gay men have something in common – loving people of the same sex – and are to varying degrees punished for it. This creates an important experience of solidarity and friendship which has manifested itself particularly clearly in the AIDS crisis. Yet there are vital differences between gay men and lesbians. Although gay men are dangerous anomalies under patriarchy, the fact that they are men guarantees them privilege over most women, most of the time. Gay men tend therefore to be seeking simply a place at the table of equality with heterosexual men and define their liberation purely in terms of sexual expression. Gay men are as capable of virulent misogyny as heterosexual men. This is, of course, a gross generalization but it points to at least a partial truth. Lesbian women as the refugees of patriarchy have been more concerned with working to overturn the table rather than join it, recognising that the complex interplay of forces are building perpetual injustice. We have tended to see our liberation in terms of relationship rather than sexual expression. (*Just Good Friends*, pp. 22–3)

William Lindsey acknowledges the point Stuart is making:

In linking homophobia to misogyny, I do not by any means wish to deny that gay men are incapable of adopting misogynistic positions. One must ask, for example, if resistance to women's aspirations to justice within the structures of some churches (as in the women's ordination movement) is fueled by a misogyny that receives the support of gay priests. ('The AIDS crisis and the Church', pp. 28–9, footnote 33)

Although I use the term 'homosexuality' quite often in this book, I have tried to remember that one reason why the experience of lesbian women is radically different from that of gay men is due to the fact that, being women, they too are affected by the oppressive influence of patriarchy on the lives of all women. I am also conscious of the fact that, in the context of HIV/AIDS, it would be very misleading to give the impression that gays and lesbians are equally at risk of HIV infection. Too often it has been assumed that there is no significance difference in the way lesbians and gays are experiencing the AIDS pandemic. Nevertheless, HIV infection is certainly a serious concern for lesbians, even though there is still considerable debate with regard to possible modes of transmission (cf. Berer, Marge with Ray, Sunanda eds., *Women and HIV/AIDS: an International Resource Book*, London, Pandora, 1993, p. 117).

A DISTURBING QUESTION: DOES THE CHRISTIAN STANCE ON HOMOSEXUALITY HELP TO SPREAD HIV/AIDS?

Some years ago, in an article on Charles Curran in *The Times* (30 August 1986), I wrote:

The approach I am describing would say that if some men and women are homosexual in a deep, almost constitutional way, that does not make them any the less persons loved by God and called to live lives of interpersonal love. Being a homosexual does not automatically bring with it a vocation to celibacy. The Gospel is hardly 'good news' to such a person if he or she is told by the Church: 'As a person you are loved by God but the capacity you have for loving at this very deep level of your personal being is displeasing to God.' This approach is simply saying that in some way or other the Church must help homosexuals to live lives of faithful love.

I went on to suggest that our Christian teaching on homosexuality might be contributing to the spread of HIV/AIDS since it left many gays feeling isolated and confused. It did not encourage them to form faithful partnerships. That concern is still felt by many, myself included. That is why, in this chapter, I will be exploring whether the current Catholic teaching on homosexuality does justice to the best theological thinking of our day. Perhaps respect for our living Christian tradition should be leading us not merely to tolerate homosexual relationships as some kind of compromise or 'lesser of two evils', but actually to celebrate the goodness of faithful loving homosexual relationships and recognize them as 'sacraments' of God's loving presence among us.

If this position is sustainable, not only will the Gospel be heard as 'good news' by such gays and lesbians but the whole Church will surely be the richer for it. Of course, I will not be denying that the Gospel is a two-edged sword and challenges unlove and selfishness in all our lives. Hence, I will also be facing the disturbing truth that the Gospel presents a healing and life-giving challenge in the face of any unlove or selfishness disfiguring and wounding the lives of gays and lesbians or impoverishing their lifestyle. However, this healing challenge of the Gospel applies equally to non-gay Christians and their Churches. I would not want to assume that all woundedness found among gays and lesbians is self-inflicted. I have no doubt that at least some of it is Church-inflicted!

In his book *AIDS, Gays, and the American Catholic Church* (Cleveland, OH, The Pilgrim Press, 1994), Richard L. Smith explores the social construction of homosexuality and its impact on how HIV/AIDS has been perceived. He quotes one writer, Kevin Gordon, as saying, 'Like a blotter AIDS has absorbed old, attached, pre-constructed, long-buried associations between sex and sin, sin and death' (p. 18). Smith himself maintains that 'our metaphors for AIDS have been constructed, to a large extent, out of our inherited cultural metaphors for homosexuality'. That is why he believes it is necessary to undertake 'a critical examination of the historical processes that have yielded our current religious, scientific, and popular metaphors for homosexuality in order to shed some light on the ways in which they have influenced our understandings of AIDS' (p. 19). What the Churches have taught about homosexuality in the light of their general approach to sexual ethics has been a very influential part of this process of social construction. However, attitudes are beginning to change and this is partly due to the way HIV/AIDS has touched the Christian community.

LEARNING FROM EXPERIENCE

The presence of HIV/AIDS in the gay community has forced Christian Churches into closer contact with gays and with some of the groups who make up the gay community. For the most part, Christian Churches had tended to marginalize gays and lesbians and had condemned same-sex relationships and expressions of same-sex love. This had created a wide divide between the Churches and the gay community. However, once HIV/AIDS entered the gay scene, two pastoral principles led individual Christians, and the Churches as a whole, to come into much closer contact with gays and the gay community.

The first was the Gospel emphasis on caring for the sick. In New Testament times those who were sick tended to be marginalized by 'respectable' society who believed there was some kind of causal link between illness and sin. Jesus challenged this mentality. Consequently, the sick seem to have been drawn to him like a magnet. It is especially noticeable that contact with lepers seems to have played a major part in the healing ministry of Jesus. In our own day Christians who have felt themselves drawn to care for people living with HIV/AIDS believe that they should show the same compassion to people living with HIV/AIDS as Jesus did to the lepers of his day.

However, often their own feelings and criticism from some of their fellow Christians have made them face the question: 'In caring for gays living with HIV/AIDS am I giving implicit approval to their gay lifestyle?' This question becomes all the more pressing when such caring involves close contact with the gay partner who is usually the principal carer and is supporting the sick person by intimate expressions of love and tenderness. This is where the second element of Christian wisdom, 'Hate the sin, but love the sinner' has provided reassurance to these Christian carers. What they are doing is caring for this sick person here and now. The cause of the sickness, even if thought to be self-inflicted, is irrelevant. They even remind themselves that many other forms of terminal illness, lung cancer, for instance, can in particular instances be self-inflicted due to the sufferer's lifestyle. Yet no one would suggest that such people should be outside Christian care and compassion.

This kind of approach has provided the main thrust to many statements on HIV/AIDS emanating from official Church sources. Bishops urged Christians to be compassionate to all infected with HIV/AIDS. They stressed the need for carers to be non-judgemental. How a person had become infected was irrelevant to the human care and compassion called for in their present time of need. For instance, the late Cardinal Bernardin wrote:

> From a moral point of view, we do not approve of certain sexual activities through which AIDS can be transmitted, and we must be very clear about encouraging people to live in accordance with the church's moral code. We teach what is morally right and wrong. But when a person has AIDS, then we are nonjudgmental. The person may or may not have contracted the disease through an immoral action or behaviour. We treat AIDS as a human disease, and we reach out to the person with compassion. We do not ask how he or she contracted the disease. (quoted in Richard L. Smith, *AIDS, Gays, and the American Catholic Church*, p. 85)

However, that is not the end of the story. Something else was happening among the Christian carers and even among the community at large, including the Christian Churches. They were being brought into contact with the gay partners of the men they were caring for. They discovered that these gay men were caring for their sick and dying partners with an extraordinarily dedicated and faithful love and care. This had a very powerful impact on these Christian carers. Believing in the presence of God's loving Spirit within human life they could not but be moved by this striking phenomenon. They felt they were experiencing the deep human goodness of the love of these gay partners. As Christians, their incarnational faith told them that in this human love they were witnessing God's gracious love in action. They were in the presence of something good and holy. Quite literally, in many cases this was a revelation to them. This experience is noted in the report of the working party *On the Theology of Marriage* presented to the 1994 General Assembly of the Church of Scotland:

> Many gay and lesbian partners do seek and intend permanent commitment, some with explicit understanding of their relationship as God-given and God-sustained . . . (This) will not seem so

strange to those who have witnessed the real love and caring which exist in many homosexual partnerships. Thos who have stood in a pastoral relationship to the early victims of AIDS have often been humbled by the devoted cherishing exhibited by the partners of the patients (although these same partners are sometimes completely ignored in their bereavement and denied even a mention at their loved one's funeral). (9.1)

Richard L. Smith also gives some examples of this drawn from his interviews with Catholic carers in two archdioceses in the USA. He reports one minister as saying:

AIDS has opened a door between gay people and the church. It gives a lot of people in the church an excuse, a safe avenue to work in the gay community without being labeled. AIDS has been an agent prompting reflection on sexuality . . . They see heroism and selfless activity in the gay community. They come to ask: How could this be bad? How could this be what the church is telling us it is? (*AIDS, Gays and the American Catholic Church*, p. 94)

Another interviewee says something similar when asked what he would like to say to the Pope in the light of his experience of caring for people living with AIDS:

I could put my message into one word: Listen. Listen to people's stories so that we can discover the sacred in them. The difficulty I have with the church and the hierarchy is a positive inability to listen to people's stories, so they're not dealing with a movement I believe to be of God's spirit. (p. 94)

In general, Smith found that these carers, some of them clergy who are themselves gay, have constructed from their own caring experience an understanding of HIV/AIDS and homosexuality significantly different from that of the bishops:

I would regard all the men and women I spoke with as 'gay-positive', that is, as regarding homosexuality as a normal variant of human sexuality in general. While maintaining some critical perspectives on gay culture, they nevertheless understand being gay as a legitimate and healthy sexual identity . . . Unlike the bishops, they are *not* of the opinion that AIDS results from immoral behaviour. They do not see its remedy as a simple return to a traditional sexual ethic. Moreover, they do not find it necessary, as they provide a rationale for their ministry, benignly to disregard the fact that a given client might be gay and in a relationship with a person of the same sex; on the contrary, they see such relationships as calling for affirmation and respect. In these ways, these ministers are operating from a world-view that is different from that of the bishops. Consequently, . . . their construction of AIDS is noticeably different as well. (p. 91)

Naturally, this picture of gay partners' faithful love and care for their lovers with AIDS was not true in every case. Even when it was true, it should not be idealized. Like all love, there was the natural struggle and tension involved in such a time of stress. Yet even its very vulnerability was perceived as a striking feature of its strength. Moreover, the part of this experience which was so challenging to Christian carers was not just the love and fidelity of the caring partner. It was also the response of the sick partner to this love. Its impact seemed to be truly life-giving, even in the very process of dying. They did not resign themselves simply to dying with AIDS. They lived positively with AIDS even during the long process of their dying. It seemed to be the mutual love of their gay partnership which empowered this positive approach to death. Often even the funeral of the dead partner was a powerful celebration of life and hope. Such funerals could offer an inspiring challenge to the unimaginative and impersonal liturgies occasionally experienced at some Catholic funerals.

It should be noted, too, that it was not only the love and devotion of partners in the midst of AIDS that made a deep impression on many Christians. It was also the way the gay community as a whole rallied round its sick, dying and bereaved members. Their highly visible ethos of collective and mutual care and concern gave the lie to many of the stereotypes of the gay community.

The place of experience as a source for theology seems self-evident to most theologians in the post-Vatican II Church. Therefore, the experience of these Christian carers is something that needs to be taken seriously by Christian theologians. It challenges the traditional Christian stance on homosexual relationships and their loving expression. Moreover, although the HIV/AIDS pandemic has been the occasion when this experience first began to have a real impact on the Churches, it must not be forgotten that the real source for theology in this area is the experience of gays themselves. In recent decades, the gay community has been coming out of the ghetto and demanding a hearing. As well as protesting against discrimination against gays and demanding equal rights in all walks of life, they have also begun to speak with pride of their own personal experience of being gay. A striking example of that is found in the Dignity Task Force document, 'Sexual ethics: experience, growth, challenge', published in *Dignity*

USA, 1989, pp. 1–16. This statement is an important theological source, even though, as I note in my review in *The Month*, 1990, pp. 368–73, it could have been more helpful and informative for those of us who are not privy to the gay experience.

FINDING THE APPROPRIATE THEOLOGICAL LANGUAGE FOR THE EXPERIENCE OF GAYS AND LESBIANS

When Christians in general began to be challenged by the 'grace-filled' experience of gay partners living lives which carried all the marks of a 'loving relationship' – and so revelatory of God – the initial reaction of theologians like myself was that this experience must be listened to. However, that initial reaction presumed that heterosexual theologians like myself would do the listening. We would examine the experience presented to us and then evaluate whether it was necessary to realign our sexual theology and ethics to take account of what we had learnt in this process.

What this overlooked was the fact that the language about homosexuality which we had all been brought up on was not adequate for expressing the positive experience of gays and lesbians. Hence, new ways of speaking about gay and lesbian experience had to be found. Initially, this could only be done by gay people themselves since it was their experience as persons which was being expressed. Moreover, what theologians like myself were failing to appreciate was that gay Christians seeking to articulate their experience are actually 'doing theology'. Finding the right language is actually part of the theological process. And that also involves looking critically at the language which has been in use but which is no longer deemed adequate. This means that Christians need to look again at the kind of theological language they use in their rejection of homosexuality and homosexual behaviour.

In particular, Christians tend to have a negative image of homosexuality and reject homosexual behaviour because they believe it is both 'not natural' and also 'condemned in the Bible'. Consequently, we need to look at those two ways of speaking.

1. The use and abuse of the language of 'natural' and 'unnatural'

It is often argued that it is 'unnatural' for two men or two women to make love to each other. That is not the 'natural' way for people to behave. The bodily make-up of human beings as sexual persons is obviously designed for the man–woman complementarity of sexual intercourse. 'Nature' has not made us for homosexual behaviour. God's purposes are written into our bodily nature. Homosexual behaviour goes against God's design and violates the way God has created us. We must respect the kind of persons God has made us to be. For anyone understanding 'natural' and 'unnatural' in this way, there is nothing more to be said.

However, as we have already seen in Chapter Two, the contemporary understanding of the traditional 'natural law' concept holds that our bodily givenness is only one dimension of our nature as human persons. Of itself, therefore, it does not provide us with any moral imperative, let alone one which is definitive and absolute. To discern what is in keeping with the good of the human person, integrally and adequately considered, we have to view our bodily givenness in the light of the other 'given' dimensions of our being human persons. To do this we have to draw on the best knowledge our contemporary culture can offer us to help us understand ourselves as human persons. To reject as immoral same-sex love relationships and the mutually acceptable and enriching bodily expression of their love simply because they are considered 'against nature' in the reductionist sense mentioned earlier hardly does justice to the Vatican II criterion of the human person, integrally and adequately considered. Our bodily dimension certainly has to be taken into account since we are our bodies. But we are also more than our bodies. We are multi-dimensional persons. What is 'natural' for us humanly and theologically can only be understood by looking at the wider context of our multidimensional richness. In that wider context it might well be possible to use the language of what is 'natural' to express the positive goodness of the experience of gay men and lesbian women. As we shall see in the next chapter, that is precisely what some Christian Church documents have done.

It is worth noting that Andrew Sullivan, in his book *Virtually Normal: An Argument about Homosexuality* (London, Picador, 1995), even uses this 'what is natural' language to suggest that homosexuality is part of the rich diversity of God's creation. After presenting the Church's belief that to accept the goodness of homosexuality would be 'to subvert the mystery at the heart of God's creation, to commit a crime against the complementary dualism of the universe', he goes on to write:

> But all these arguments are arguments for the *centrality* of heterosexual acts in nature, not their exclusiveness. It is surely possible to concur with these sentiments, even to appreciate their insight,

while also conceding that it is nevertheless true that nature seems to have provided a jagged lining to this homogeneous cloud, a spontaneously occurring contrast that could conceivably be understood to complement – even dramatize – the central male–female order . . . so the homosexual person might be seen as a natural foil to the heterosexual norm, a variation that does not eclipse the theme, but resonates with it. Extinguishing – or prohibiting – homosexuality is, from this point of view, not a virtuous necessity, but the real crime against nature, a refusal to accept the variety of God's creation, a denial of the way in which the other need not threaten, but may actually give depth and contrast to, the self.

This . . . is, perhaps, just as consonant with the tradition of natural law as the Church's current position. It is more consonant with what seems to occur in nature; it seeks an end to every form of natural life; it upholds the dignity of each human person as made in the image of God and seeks to bring each into the human and Christian universe. It sees in the multifaceted character of God's creation reasons to accept rather than reasons to fear. It resonates too with that ancient and rich notion that one proof of God's existence is in the sheer diversity and complexity of His creation, a creation that is less to be regimented than to be marvelled at. (pp. 46–8)

2. The use and abuse of the language of God's word in the Bible

The development of a more open language in which to discuss homosexuality is also stymied by assertions that there can be nothing to discuss since homosexuality is clearly condemned in the Bible; that must close the question for Christians.

This has been a problem across the board in nearly all Christian Churches. Within the Roman Catholic Church it comes out clearly in the 1975 Congregation for the Doctrine of the Faith (CDF) *Declaration on certain questions concerning Sexual Ethics*: 'In Sacred Scripture they (homosexual acts) are condemned as a serious depravity and even presented as the sad consequence of rejecting God. This judgement of Scripture does not of course permit us to conclude that all those who suffer from this anomaly are personally responsible for it, but it does attest to the fact that homosexual acts are intrinsically disordered and can in no case be approved of' (n. 8). The even stronger condemnation found in the 1986 CDF *Letter to the bishops of the Catholic Church on the pastoral care of homosexual persons* is based on a similar reading of biblical texts, though spelt out in more detail. Moreover, it warns against any exegesis which would call this reading into question:

> An essential dimension of authentic pastoral care is the identification of causes of confusion regarding the Church's teaching. One is a new exegesis of Sacred Scripture which claims variously that Scripture has nothing to say on the subject of homosexuality, or that it somehow tacitly approves of it, or that all of its moral injunctions are so culture-bound that they are no longer applicable to contemporary life. These views are gravely erroneous . . . (n. 4)

Furthermore, it goes on to state that 'it is essential to recognise that the Scriptures are not properly understood when they are interpreted in a way which contradicts the Church's living Tradition. To be correct, the interpretation of Scripture must be in substantial accord with that Tradition' (n. 5). This is tantamount to a virtual checkmate if the CDF claims the authority to interpret precisely what constitutes that tradition!

The Methodist Church, too, has found the way forward blocked by arguments based on biblical exegesis. An official Working Party produced a major report in 1980, *A Christian Understanding of Human Sexuality*. It formulated conclusions which offered the possibility of a more positive evaluation of stable homosexual relations and their physical expression (cf. nn.18 & 20). However, the Working Party was clearly divided on the issue of homosexuality in the Bible and the impact of biblical ethics on present-day Christian moral teaching. Two different approaches to biblical interpretation were present among the members. These are spelt out in an Appendix which is almost as long as the report itself. Conference referred the report to the Districts and Circuits for study and evaluation.

The message came back from the pews that one of the two issues most troubling people was 'the place of Scripture in the formulation of moral guidance'. Accordingly, the revised report presented in 1982 contained an excellent section on 'The place of Scripture and Tradition' (nn. 2–18). Once again, the Working Party's conclusion represented a division of opinion, even though the majority were clearly in favour of a more positive acceptance:

> (50) . . . The recognition that many people are homosexual by nature, and that they are as capable as other people of full Christian discipleship and of deeply loving and committed relationships with each other has been changing the climate of

Christian opinion in the last decade or so. The Working Party therefore records its unanimous judgement that there is no reason to deny the right of those who are homosexually oriented to be members, office holders, local preachers or ministers of the Church. (But it differs in its judgement about homosexual practices as is made clear in the following two paragraphs.)

(51) Some Christians hold on grounds of either Scripture or tradition, or both, that homosexuality is a defect or handicap and should never be given physical expression, but rather channelled or sublimated into creative activities such as the caring professions or the arts.

(52) Other Christians, including a majority of the Working Party, recognise such creative possibilities, but hold on the basis of their understanding of Scripture and on other grounds that heterosexual and homosexual relationships alike are to be valued according to the presence or absence of love as the New Testament describes it. They agree that for some homosexual people (as for some heterosexual people) celibacy is a vocation, and that for others a choice between a partnership without physical expression and one that includes genital expression within a committed relationship is to be accepted as a choice which Christians may responsibly make.

Once again Conference did not feel it could make any definitive judgement and directed the Division of Social Responsibility to have the report studied and discussed throughout the Church.

The debate simmered on until 1990 when a further report, entitled *Report of Commission on Human Sexuality*, was presented to Conference. Like the previous two reports, this one ran aground on the same issue of the use of the Bible in the discussion of contemporary moral issues: 'there were differences of opinion, judgement and conviction within the Commission about the way in which Scripture should be used in this exercise, and about its value and authority relative to contemporary experience' (n. 100).

Other Churches display similar deep differences of opinion regarding the legitimate use of Scripture in discussing the issue of homosexuality. In his World Council of Churches (WCC) study guide, *Living in Covenant with God and One Another* (Geneva, WCC Publications, 1990), Robin Smith compares two contrasting statements on homosexuality, one from the Reformed Church of America and the other from the Uniting Church of Australia. He concludes that their divergence of view demonstrates that 'one's attitude to homosexuality is greatly influenced by how one interprets the Bible' (p. 108). Clearly, within many Christian Churches opinion is very divided about how the Bible can be understood as offering moral guidance for Christian gays and lesbians today.

Aquinas was a great believer in the principle, *non nomina sed argumenta*. In other words, we move towards the truth by the quality of our theological arguments rather than by a head-count of theologians. In the light of my fairly extensive reading of Church documents on homosexuality, it seems clear to me that the above two different positions found among Christians and documented in various official reports cannot be judged to have equal intrinsic authority at the level of biblical exegesis and theological scholarship. The view which leaves open a more positive approach to homosexual relationships and their expression seems to be an interpretation which is based on the best of modern textual exegesis, taking fully into account the historical and cultural contexts of the relevant biblical passages. And it combines this with a more satisfactory approach to the knotty problem of how far ethical norms found in the Bible can leap across the cultural gap of twenty centuries and have a bearing on the contemporary moral questions we have to wrestle with in our post-modern age. Though the opposite view is held with great conviction by many Christians in different Churches, the weakness of its biblical and theological justification is becoming increasingly recognized among biblical scholars and theologians across the Churches.

However, that does not mean that the Bible has no inspired guidance for gay and lesbian Christians. A helpful summary of this guidance is given by the eminent Methodist scripture scholar, Victor Paul Furnish. He ends a masterly paper, entitled 'Homosexual practices in biblical perspective', with the following conclusion:

> The church must attend to the witness of Scripture as it seeks to discern the will of God in the matter of homosexuality. Scripture provides access to the apostolic witness, wherein the believing community finds the norm by which appropriately *christian* faith and conduct, including sexual conduct, may be ascertained.
>
> It would be a simple matter if this norm could be found in what Scripture provides by way of specific rules, teachings, and advisories concerning homoerotic relationships. But that is not the case. However pertinent they may have been for the various times and circumstances within which they were originally formulated, the biblical injunctions and teachings on this topic presume much than can no longer be presumed about human

sexuality. It is certainly true that our present understanding of homosexuality is incomplete and undergoing constant revision. Yet our knowledge of this subject is vastly superior to that available in ancient Israel and the early church. Moreover, we can appreciate the complexity of the issue, as well the incompleteness of our understanding of it, in a way that the ancient world could not.

Therefore, it is not what 'the Bible says' about homoerotic relationships that constitutes the witness of Scripture to the church on this topic. Rather, in this instance as in every other the witness of Scripture is that human existence, like the whole of creation, is the gift of an omnipotent, just, benevolent, and caring God; that God's purposes are shaped and accomplished by God's love, over which nothing in all creation (including humanity's rebellious-ness) can finally prevail; that the people of God are repeatedly summoned to walk in the same love from and in which, by God's grace, they properly 'live and move and have their being'; that the claim inherent in God's love is no less boundless than the gift; and that it is in Christ that women and men of faith will find, at last, both the saving power of God's gift of love and the strength to follow where it leads. (in John J. Carey, ed., *The Sexuality Debate in North American Churches, 1988–1995: Controversies, Unresolved Issues, Future Prospects*, Lewiston, New York, Edwin Mellen Press, 1995, pp. 253–81, at pp. 272–3)

There is also no doubt that the ethical thrust in both Old and New Testaments lies in the direction of bringing justice and liberation for those whose human dignity is diminished or violated by structures of power in society which create relationships of injustice. In past centuries we were blind to how this teaching challenged the institution of slavery. As we saw in the previous chapter, today we are beginning to recognize that it challenges the structured injustices against women in society in general and in the sexual area in particular. Now we are also being asked to face a similar challenge with regard to the injustice against lesbian women and gay men which is endemic in a sexual ethics which demands that they believe that their capacity for love is an objective disorder and not a gift which they can feel both proud of and grateful to God for.

TOWARDS A GAY AND LESBIAN THEOLOGY AND SPIRITUALITY: WOUNDEDNESS AND HEALING

In Chapter Two we noted that a natural law approach which focuses solely on the doctrine of creation and by-passes the doctrine of redemption would be seriously flawed. As Nicholas Lash put it so strikingly, 'the world's forgiveness is creation's finishing' (*Believing Three Ways in God*, London, SCM, 1992, p. 119). Hence, a gay and lesbian theology and spirituality will need to face the reality of sin. Our discussion of social construction in Chapter Two makes us aware that, here too, we are dealing with a social construct which will inevitably be affected by institutional sin in a whole variety of ways. Michael Ruse, in his book *Homosexuality: A Philosophical Enquiry* (Oxford, Basil Blackwell, 1988), writes that 'If the majority stop thinking of homosexuality as a handicap and as something unpleasant, and if they stop hating homosexuals, then if nothing else we shall get a rise in the self-image of presently troubled homosexuals' (p. 215). He makes a similar point in his final conclusion: 'If . . . we treat homosexuals like normal people, then perhaps to our surprise we shall find that they are normal people' (p. 267). Ruse implies that the Church has a role to play in this: 'Here, obviously, is a place where the moral leader must work to redirect the gut feelings of the man in the street' (p. 265).

If HIV/AIDS is challenging the Church to reconsider its understanding of homosexuality and its ethical norms flowing from this understanding, in Lash's terms this could be part of the Church's seeking forgiveness. It could also mean that the Church might have an important role to play in the forgiveness of society in general *vis-à-vis* homosexuality. The result of such healing and forgiveness might be the elaboration for gay Christians of a positive spirituality which starts from their dignity as homosexual persons and which also does justice to their need precisely as gay people for loving relationships.

Though probably not intended, there could be an opening for this development in *The Catechism of the Catholic Church* (London, Geoffrey Chapman, 1994). Homosexuality is considered under the general heading, *The Vocation to Chastity*. Here chastity is presented very positively as 'the successful integration of sexuality within the person and thus the inner unity of man in his bodily and spiritual being' (n. 2337). After insisting that 'the virtue of chastity blossoms in *friendship*', the Catechism goes on to say that 'Chastity is expressed notably in *friendship with one's neighbour*. Whether it develops between persons of the same or opposite sex, friendship represents a great good for all. It leads to spiritual communion' (n. 2347).

It is significant that homosexuality is given a sub-section all of its own with the heading, *Chastity and homosexuality* (nn. 2357–2359) and is not even mentioned in the sub-section, *Offences against chastity* (nn. 2351–2356). Sadly but not surprisingly, homosexual acts are described as 'intrinsically disordered', though there is no repetition of the CDF's statement on the disorder of the homosexual orientation itself. Moreover, the final two paragraphs contain much that is positive *vis-à-vis* homosexuality.

A much more promising opening for the development of a more positive spirituality of homosexual relationships is found in Cardinal Hume's *A Note on the Teaching of the Catholic Church Concerning Homosexual People* (February 1995, revised in April 1997). While accepting the Church's teaching that 'homosexual genital acts are objectively wrong', the Cardinal goes on to write:

> (8) Friendship is a gift from God. Friendship is a way of loving. Friendship is necessary for every person. To equate friendship and full sexual involvement with another is to distort the very concept of friendship. Sexual loving presupposes friendship but friendship does not require full sexual involvement. It is a mistake to say or think or presume that if two persons of the same or different sexes enjoy a deep and lasting friendship then they must be sexually involved.

> (9) Love between two persons, whether of the same sex or of a different sex, is to be treasured and respected. 'Jesus loved Martha and her sister and Lazarus', we read. (Jn 11,5) When two persons love they experience in a limited manner in this world what will be their unending delight when one is with God in the next. To love another is in fact to reach out to God who shares his lovableness with one we love. To be loved is to receive a sign, or a share, of God's unconditional love.

> (10) To love another, whether of the same sex or of a different sex, is to have entered the area of the richest human experience. But that experience of love is spoiled, whether it is in marriage or in friendship, when we do not think and act as God wills us to think and act. Human loving is precarious for human nature is wounded and frail. Thus marriage and friendship will never be easy to handle. We shall often fail, but the ideal remains.

It is interesting to note that Cardinal Hume, like the Catechism, focuses on friendship. He sees it as 'a gift from God' and 'a way of loving'. The Roman Catholic theologian, Elizabeth Stuart, herself a lesbian, in her very thought-provoking book *Just Good Friends: Towards a Lesbian and Gay*

Theology of Relationships, takes the notion of 'friendship' and makes it the lynch-pin of her sexual ethics. The starting point of her presentation is a combination of her own experience as a lesbian woman and her listening to and interpreting the experience of other lesbian women – and gay men, too. I shall return to her presentation in a later chapter. For the present, it is sufficient to note that Stuart's book fulfils the hope expressed earlier that lesbian women and gay men should express the positive goodness of lesbian and gay relationships and loving in a language which is comprehensible to the rest of us who are not gay or lesbian. Her book is a fine example of 'theology from within'. She expresses the importance of this in her preface:

> if we really do believe that human beings are made in the image and likeness of God then when we seek to do theology around certain people's lives our first duty is to go to them and listen to the way that they make sense of the experience of God in their lives. It is not simply a matter of receiving evidence from them, as some church bodies have begun to do in connection with homosexuality. It is about giving priority to their theology as the people who know most about the subject and have to live it every moment of their lives. (pp. xvii–xviii)

As Xavier John Seubert notes in his excellent article, 'The sacramentality of metaphors: reflections on homosexuality', in *Cross Currents*, Spring 1991, pp. 52–68, this kind of work needs to be accepted gratefully by the Church as a rich contribution to its ongoing commitment to the truth. Of course, that does not imply uncritical acceptance of everything that is said. Nevertheless, without the kind of theological reflection and writing of people like Elizabeth Stuart, there is no possibility of real dialogue on this issue in the Church. And without dialogue we cannot claim to be respecting our commitment to the truth. Seubert puts this well:

> The Christian moral tradition stresses the primacy of conscience. I translate this to mean that an individual's experience of the truth must be respected. Truth does not consist simply in formulated norms by which reality is judged. It is also found in the way the whole human person responds to a reality in those cases where any other response would falsify the existence of that reality. In the case of homosexuality, a significant group of Christians calls upon the broader church to look with them at their experience of the truth of their reality. Their request cannot be dismissed or prejudged by norms that have not been informed by anything like their experience.

What is needed, first of all, is a continuation of the meta-
phorical process. Metaphors must be developed to include the
richest possibilities of gay and lesbian life. This will demand
that gays and lesbians within the church further articulate
the goodness of their lives as gays and lesbians and relate that
goodness to their lives as Christians.

The prevalent metaphors have not been informed by
what many gays and lesbians consider to be homosexuality's
potential for human dignity and fulfilment. Until the homosexual
experience is truthfully spoken and respectfully heard, the church
will be unable to stand in the truth, endure it, and live from it.
(pp. 62–3)

In his Foreword to Smith's *AIDS, Gays and the American Catholic Church*,
Robert N. Bellah writes:

A principled rejection of gay sexuality, whether put forward by the
church or any other sector of society, is morally indefensible. It has
the same status today as arguments for the inferiority of women.
To remain stuck in that position, as the church for the time being
seems likely to do, is not only unfortunate: it makes the church
collaborate in continuing forms of domination. To put it even
more strongly: it makes the church collaborate in sin. (pp. xii–xiii)

Of course, a person-centred base for a positive gay and lesbian
theology will not give an ethical *carte blanche* for any and every kind of
conduct among lesbians and gay men. It would be an affront to their
dignity to suggest that their behaviour should not be governed by the
normal rules of human decency, justice and respect for persons. As
mentioned earlier, to present the Gospel positively as genuine 'good
news' for gay men and lesbians does not mean that the Gospel does
not challenge them to eradicate from their lives whatever violates the
dignity of persons or is destructive of personal and social relationships.

We are all of us, heterosexuals and gays and lesbians alike, wounded
people. However, because lesbians and gay men have been the victims
of seriously oppressive social stigmatization and injustice, it is possible
that for some of them at least this woundedness will have had an
adverse effect on their sense of self-worth, their integration of sexual
identity and their ability to form deep and lasting relationships. Of
course, many heterosexual persons share these same problems but it is
possible that they are experienced much more severely by some gays
and lesbians due to the extra social pressures working against them.
As Michael Ruse has pointed out (cf. *Homosexuality*, pp. 10–11), the

healing of this woundedness needs to go hand in hand with the healing of the woundedness of homophobia which is so widespread both in Church and in society.

To the extent that such woundedness shows in the behaviour of some gay men and women and even in the collective behaviour in some gay and lesbian communities, healing is only possible to the extent that the woundedness of their behaviour is recognized and owned by the gays and lesbians involved. Such healing diagnosis needs to be based on agreed criteria for distinguishing 'healthy' behaviour from 'wounded' behaviour. Part of a more open dialogue towards a positive spirituality for homosexual persons will surely need to have on its agenda how to discern what kinds of homosexual behaviour are abusive of persons rather than expressive of genuine love or preventing growth in emotional maturity rather than developing the capacity to sustain faithful loving relationships.

Not being homosexual myself and recognizing that the heterosexual scene has more than its share of negative behaviour, including the whole patriarchal scenario, I hesitate to express my own negative reaction to certain aspects of the gay scene paraded on the media or given a high profile in some public demonstrations. Nevertheless, I suspect that there is something here which should not be brushed under the carpet. Matthew Fox in his very positive article on 'The spiritual journey of the homosexual . . . and just about everybody else' tackles this point directly, though without passing any moral condemnation of the individuals involved. Noting that 'the pain and suffering that a homosexual in a homophobic culture undergoes can be either redemptive or alienating', he goes on to comment on the second possibility:

> When, however, for any number of reasons a homosexual cannot pass through the pain that homophobic cultures rain on him or her, then a psychospiritual arrest can happen and the homosexual becomes a scapegoat, a self-fulfilling prophecy of a homophobic society, a broken and essentially lonely person who, in his or her alienation, truly feels like an alien, a stranger in a sick society. In the alien's effort to please that society he or she falls prey to its own worst sins: power over, power under, sadomasochism, consumerism, hatred of the body, inability to sustain relationships, adolescent arrest, and egoistic quests for perfectionism and immortality. Like the slave who has imbibed the ideology of his slave master, the homosexual then fulfils the prophecy of the heterosexual, plays out the worst stereotypes of the repressed

homophobic conscience, and gives to the sexist homophobic society a weapon of great strength: 'See,' he will say, 'what I warned you about the homosexual.' (in Robert Nugent, ed., *A Challenge to Love: Gay and Lesbian Catholics in the Church*, New York, Crossroad, 1989, pp. 189–204, at p. 190)

These might seem hard and challenging words, but they come from a theologian who, a few lines earlier, had made his own the experience-based words of a sister retreat-director who said that 'the people she encountered who were "the most beautiful Christians of all" were very often homosexual men and women' (p. 189).

In his article, 'The homosexual revolution and hermeneutics', in *Concilium* (no. 173, pp. 55–64), John Coleman notes that the gay community has, for the most part, shown itself capable of self-criticism (p. 62). After quoting most of the passage from Fox given above, he goes on to mention how many in the women's movement are critical of gay pornography. They also believe that 'homosexual glorification of youth and the beautiful body similar to the prevalent attitudes toward women in modern societies . . . too easily fixates erotic interest in an alienating process of impersonalisation by making the object of sexual interest a mere *object*' (p. 62). Coleman adds the wise observation that it is these pathologies which should 'command the best moral efforts of gays'. In other words, tackling them should be an important part of the self-healing process.

I am conscious of being rather out of my depth here. While editing this chapter, I received an e-mail from a friend overseas, telling me of the AIDS-related death of a gay priest whose ministry had been largely among the gay community and those affected by HIV/AIDS. It is worth quoting some of my friend's letter:

B died peacefully at noon yesterday in the hospital where he had assisted in so many deaths on the AIDS floor. Someone should write his biography. Last year, for instance, he told me about ministering to S, a 25-year old drug addict and prostitute before he died. S had striking good looks and a career as a model. He was thrown out of his 'loving' Catholic family at sixteen because he was gay. He got into the drug scene and quickly contracted AIDS. By the time B met him his good looks were savaged by Kaposi's sarcoma. Penniless and homeless, B found him temporary accommodation at a presbytery. After S died, B fulfilled his dying wish by travelling up north with his ashes to bury him with family. The family wanted a requiem but no public acknowledgement of how he had died. The funeral was a very lonely affair with S's family openly hostile to a group of gay bikers who turned up on their Harleys to pay respects. B said the official funeral and interment was alien to S with no acknowledgement of his real life.

The real celebration took place afterwards, minus the family, in a gay bar much frequented by S in his lifetime. With much laughter, song, booze and tears, the gay community celebrated S's life. A drag artist performed 'for S' a song that he always loved. B described the church service as prim, dead and not at all hope-filled. In contrast, the liturgy in the pub – the drag queens, the much-tattooed bikers, and the rich assortment of what S's parents would characterise as 'low life' – showed how much S had been loved and appreciated. It was very 'hope-filled' too. B said that the family hardly shed a tear. Yet all evening at the pub people broke down and held each other and wept, showing how much S had been loved by his gay family.

While I believe that theology has to make faith-sense of experience, to borrow a phrase from Jack Mahoney, I could not begin to try to unpack the theological significance of that very challenging piece of experience. Nevertheless, I believe that there is much to be learnt from it and similar experiences. It might, for instance, be saying something to us about the possibility of an individual who is emotionally deprived and developmentally immature being capable of profound personal moral goodness. To that extent, it might be linked to some of the points developed in Chapter Seven. But it might also be saying something to us about the need for those of us who are not gay or lesbian to listen to and try to understand more the difference between our experience and that of our gay brothers and lesbian sisters. As a lesbian friend wrote to me recently: 'The Church is (in part) gay and lesbian and so, in reflecting on homosexuality, it is reflecting on its own being.'

In his Foreword to Smith's *AIDS, Gays and the American Catholic Church*, referred to above, Robert Bellah offers some cautionary advice on this reflective process. After remarking that the experience of those in care ministry in the area of AIDS 'needs intelligent theological and ethical reflection, not simple affirmation', he goes on to say:

> It will not do to substitute expressive individualism for unreflec-tive moralism, and that is a real temptation in the gay community . . . But a genuine attention to the lived reality of gay life in contemporary America is the essential starting point for any reflection that would put it in the context of a Christian form of life. (p. xiii)

Bellah also offers a note of warning. Even if a characteristic of the age we are living in is 'an effort to make a great moral advance, to overcome structures of domination that have characterised human societies for millennia' (p. xi) – and he highlights as most striking 'the struggle for the equality of women with men' in this connection – another characteristic of our age is more morally questionable:

> The challenge to previously accepted ways of structuring the relation between dominant and subordinate groups has gone hand in hand with the challenge to normative order itself. Individual freedom, which, rightly understood, is certainly a noble cause, has been used as an argument for the abandonment of such traditional virtues as loyalty and responsibility, undermining commitment to spouse, friends, and community. If traditional structures were oppressive there is the temptation to abandon structures altogether, with chaotic consequences. The American gay community has certainly been caught up in this movement of moral liberation on the one hand and anarchy on the other. (p. xi)

Bellah's warning will be kept in mind in Chapter Six when, under the rubric of the 'pro-freedom' characteristic of positive Christian sexual ethics, we look at the freedom of the human person and its essential link with relational and social responsibility. Despite the above warning, Bellah insists that this should not divert the Church from a whole-hearted involvement in the struggle against the structures of domination. However, it should alert the Church to discern where its priorities lie in this struggle:

> The church is under no obligation to affirm the antinomian tendencies of our culture, gay or otherwise. Rather it should undertake the difficult task of attempting to create a context of love and moral responsibility for homosexual relationships as for heterosexual ones . . . Creating such a persuasive ideal is what the problem is and that is where the energy of the church should be going. (p. xiii)

The fact that I share the same conviction is one of the main reasons why I am stepping in where angels fear to tread in attempting to write this book!

A couple of gay and lesbian friends to whom I showed a draft of this chapter commented that I tend to imply that 'good' gay men and lesbians should behave like 'good' heterosexual people. One of them wrote: 'There is a tinge of gay and lesbian sexuality being accept-able if the difference between homosexuality and heterosexuality is minimized!' Far from wanting to minimize the difference, I am trying to work on the assumption that both these sexual orientations are different ways of being human sexual persons. I am utterly convinced that there are not two Gospel moralities, one for heterosexuals and one for gays and lesbians. I believe that the fundamental Christian human values and virtues apply equally to heterosexuals and to gays and lesbians, even though the precise way in which they are made flesh in real life will be affected by a person's sexual orientation. Moreover, sexual orientation is precisely that, an 'orientation', not a totally different form of sexuality. Consequently, I cannot accept that there is a fundamentally different sexual ethic for gays and lesbians. Scientific evidence seems to support the assumption of the 1982 Methodist Working Party report that '(homosexual persons) are as capable as other people . . . of deeply loving and committed relationships with each other' (n. 50, cf. pp. 75–6 above). The Christian approach to homosexuality argued in this book is obviously based on the same assumption. It also rejects as untrue the many 'myths' about homo-sexuality (e.g. that homosexual persons tend to be paedophiles). There seems to be no scientific evidence to support such myths (cf. below, pp. 161–2).

Sexuality is a dimension to our being human persons which we all share, even though it is modified by our sexual orientation. As a Christian, I believe that this sexual dimension is an important aspect of our being made persons in the image of a relational, loving and life-giving God. We are most true to ourselves as sexual human persons, therefore, to the extent that we realize the potentiality of our sexuality by going out to each other in love, by joyfully expressing that love in a way which is appropriate to the character and depth of our relationships and by contributing to the life-giving enterprise of receiving our human existence as gift and accepting our responsibility to prepare a future worth passing on to future generations.

Joy and pleasure are part of that scenario but only in so far as they belong within the humanly rich context of interpersonal relationships. Outside of that context and pursued purely for their own sake, they do not seem to do justice to who we are as relational persons. I recognize that there is no way I can tease out what all this means in practice for gay men and lesbians. That is why I want to be open to learning from them how our common Christian sexual ethics is to be understood in a way which does justice to their experience as gays and lesbians. When I try, in Chapter Six, to explore some aspects of this sexual ethics which we share in common, I hope it will be recognizable as a Christian *sexual* ethics and not just a *heterosexual* ethics.

A 'TIME OF AIDS' – A TIME FOR POSITIVE LIVING AND POSITIVE THINKING

As mentioned in the previous chapter, the Irish moral theologian, Enda McDonagh makes the point that at this point in history we are living in 'a time of AIDS'. That is a very important dimension of the context in which we have to do our theology. He uses the word 'time' in its biblical sense of *kairos*. That means a determining moment in history. Upon our response to God's call coming to us in this *kairos* will depend the fate of future generations. In the previous chapter I argued that a careful social analysis of the appalling tragedy of the HIV/AIDS pandemic could open our ears to the voice of God calling us to conversion away from the all-pervasive evils of systemic patriarchy. In that sense, the HIV/AIDS pandemic, for all its evil, could still be transformed into a moment of grace for our human family.

In this chapter, I have been suggesting something similar with regard to homosexuality and the HIV/AIDS pandemic. Lindsey begins the article I quoted earlier, 'The AIDS crisis and the church: a time to heal', by making a similar point:

> Crises call upon cultures and institutions to look more closely at those presuppositions that have dominated discourse about central cultural problematics in the past, and to refashion these givens in light of new information and new perspectives arising out of crisis. In what follows, I propose that the AIDS crisis is such a time for the church – a cross-roads, a *kairos* – in which the church must look anew at some of its most fundamental presuppositions about homosexuality. This crisis calls the church to face more adequately the ways in which its sexual ethic with regard to gay persons functions as a mask for intents and effects that may not be deliberate, but that nevertheless flow from that teaching and prevent gay people from hearing the gospel proclaimed by the church as the good news of God's salvific love for all humanity. (pp. 12–13)

I am writing these lines shortly after attending an ecumenical AIDS meeting at which at least a quarter of the Christians present were gay. Not only were they gay, they also accepted their gay sexuality as a gift from God, a gift to be lived out in tender, loving and faithful relationships with their partners. Throughout the conference they and their partners were completely at ease, as most loving heterosexual couples would be, in openly expressing their love and tenderness through kissing, hugging, holding hands and demonstrating their joy at being in each other's company. These open demonstrations of mutual affection were a visible sign of a much deeper sharing between these couples. Obviously, such loving relationships would have been entered into initially because they felt attracted to each other. Their love would have deepened as they learned to know each other at a far deeper level than physical beauty or ways of speaking, smiling, touching, and so forth. No doubt they had had to work hard at building their relationship of love with each other. That relationship would have been consolidated through a great deal of careful listening and honest speaking, being prepared to forgive and ask for forgiveness. They must have learnt to appreciate their partner's 'otherness' as well as his 'likemindedness', being prepared to make compromises in terms of time, space, interests, friends, and so on.

I have no idea whether any of these gay Christian men actually celebrated their love for each other through genital expressions of endearment. That seemed irrelevant to me, though I presume it would not have been irrelevant to them. Perhaps all that needs to be said is that, granted the goodness of their loving and faithful relationship to each other, the criteria from Christian ethics which would seem to be relevant to how they expressed their love for each other would be something like the following: Was it mutually respectful, affirming, pleasurable? Did they both experience what they were doing as an expression of mutual love without any exploitation by either of them? And, in an age of HIV/AIDS, a further criterion to be considered might be: Did it embody a responsible concern for each other's health? I suspect that no sexual expression of love, whether heterosexual or homosexual, would score 100 per cent on all those criteria. Nevertheless, they would seem to be the general criteria of most significance for love-making between any couples, whatever their sexual orientation.

For men and women who are heterosexual, a crucial factor in their moral development is the positive acceptance of themselves as sexual persons. This is part of accepting themselves as gift from God. It involves acknowledging the giftedness of their sexuality and recognizing that this God-given gift is good. Despite a chequered history in the Church's attitude to sexuality, the importance of such acceptance of oneself as a sexual person would now seem to be agreed by everyone. It is uncontroversial.

For those Christian gay men at the meeting I referred to earlier, their self-acceptance as sexual persons must have involved accepting themselves precisely as homosexual persons. This would have been crucial to their moral development. It was the only way they could accept themselves as gift from God and acknowledge that this gift is good. However, for many Christians their position would be completely unacceptable. As we have seen, the Congregation for the Doctrine of the Faith, for instance, flatly denies it. It asserts that the homosexual condition they are calling a gift from God is actually an objective disorder. In contrast to that, a collection of much more positive statements from within the Catholic community is found in Jeannine Gramick and Robert Nugent (eds), *Voices of Hope: A Collection of Positive Catholic Writings on Gay and Lesbian Issues* (New York, Center for Homophobia Education, 1995).

Most psychologists now accept that homosexuality is a variation well within the normal range of psychological function. Despite that, not a few readers might find it difficult to accept that homosexuality is a good gift of God. Perhaps they might be helped by the true story of a mother who was faced by the double revelation that her son, who was living far from home, was gay and that he was dying of AIDS. She went to visit him and was greeted warmly at the door by his lover, whom she had never even heard about. Smith, in his book *AIDS, Gays, and the American Catholic Church*, continues the story:

> She stayed several days at the bedside of her son, playing cards and watching television with him, helping with care, talking to his doctor. But despite her satisfaction in being able to share that time with him, it was obvious that she remained disturbed about her son's homosexuality. This was particularly apparent in the rigidity and coldness with which she responded whenever his lover came into the room.
>
> After a few days, she suggested to her son that it was time to call a priest, and he agreed. Shortly after arriving at the house, the priest recognized the reason behind the mother's anxiety. After praying with her and her son, he stayed for a chat. He asked her about life in the Midwest. Eventually he asked her how she had come to meet her husband, now deceased for several years. She began to reminisce about the time they first met, the hat he was wearing, the cafe they went on their first date. She talked about the bittersweet early years of their marriage, the financial struggles they endured, and the painful fact that her family had not accepted her new husband, feeling that he was somehow beneath them.
>
> As the visit continued, the priest eventually turned to the young man with AIDS. He asked him how he had come to meet his lover. Slowly, the young man began to tell his story of how they met at a

party, where they went on their first dates, hiking trips they took, and their decision finally to establish a home together.

As his mother listened to her son, a subtle miracle began to occur. She began to recognize some profound similarities in their two stories. Despite the obvious differences between them, they both seemed to be part of a universe more vast than she had previously imagined . . . She began to understand that her son had simply but truly fallen in love with another man – just as she had once fallen in love with her husband. How amazing! How wonderful! (pp. 134–5)

When I read of this incident, I was reminded of a remark made at an AIDS conference by a Jesuit priest, Dr Jon Fuller, an authority on HIV/AIDS who combines clinical practice at Boston City Hospital with his assistant professorship at Boston University School of Medicine: 'There is nothing as similar to heterosexuality as homosexuality. They are both about loving persons precisely as persons.'

Of course, to accept that being gay or lesbian can be part of the God-given giftedness of some human persons immediately raises the question of how this giftedness is to be lived out in a way which respects and promotes the dignity of human persons. In other words, it serves to remind us that when homosexuality is understood in this positive way, it becomes an important dimension of how they respond to God's call and so needs to be viewed within the general context of Christian morality. As we have seen already, this poses a challenge to our Christian sexual ethics. It is possible that a radical reappraisal might be needed if it is to be able to accommodate a positive appreciation of homosexuality. Some people may respond to this suggestion with dismay, believing that this means yet another stage in what they see as a lowering of moral standards. However, if our more positive vision of homosexuality is really true, it should follow that a sexual ethics which is able to do justice to this, should be all that more richer since it is now constructed on the basis of more comprehensive picture of the giftedness of the human person. Part of the task to be faced in Chapter Six will involve trying to discern what shape such an enriched sexual ethics is likely to take.

THE GOSPEL AS 'GOOD NEWS' FOR GAYS AND LESBIANS

The need for a positive spirituality of homosexual relationships comes out very powerfully in a TV documentary, *Better Dead than Gay*

(Channel 4, 25 July 1995), produced and directed by Christopher O'Hare. It is the true story of a devout young Christian gay man, Simon Harvey, who was found dead in his car from a suicidal over-dose after driving himself to a secluded spot in the countryside. The programme makes extensive use of his diary and of a long letter he left explaining why he killed himself. The title of the programme is based on a remark by Simon's father that the news of his son's gayness had been just as shocking as the news of his death. He went on to say that Simon might have been saved if he had met a good Christian who could have shown him that he could have been 'cured' of his gayness. O'Hare comments: 'Sadly, Simon's letters and diaries tell a very different story.'

Simon's Christian upbringing made him believe that his gayness was sinful. Consequently, he thought himself 'too filthy to continue living'. Driven by this self-disgust – 'the word, "homosexual", was an anathema to me' – he searched frantically for a cure for 'my malady'. He felt his only hope lay in being released from his homosexuality. Some of his fellow-Christians encouraged him to believe that this was a real possibility. Consequently, he visited a variety of Christian therapists and counsellors. He was prayed over in rites of deliverance and exorcism. But 'nothing happened'. A friend, Nathan Stowe, was scathing about the kind of help Simon was being offered by his Christian friends:

> They had given him a straw to clutch on to that didn't actually exist. You cannot just wave a magic wand and make somebody gay straight . . . It's in them. They are their own person . . . It is not an illness. You are just gay and that is it . . . He was dragged off out of his depth. They drowned him in rubbish . . . They were basically saying: 'Be with us and you will be happy, you will be straight, you will be normal.' They drowned him. He didn't commit suicide. He drowned.

Near the end of the programme a Baptist minister, Robert Amess, who had been helpful to Simon earlier in his life, remarked: 'God meets us where we are'. Christopher O'Hare concluded the programme with his own very powerful comment on that remark:

> Simon didn't kill himself because he was gay or a Christian or both. Simon killed himself because he and others thought that he should not be who he was. The Christian Church says, 'Love the sinner: hate the sin'. But how can any person find self-worth and dignity without the right to express love, free of shame and

guilt. Simon's life and death are a testimony to the importance of accepting and living with difference in other people and in oneself.

Given a more positive Christian spirituality of homosexuality, Simon might well be alive today.

Tragically, Simon is not the only gay person to commit suicide. Some recent as yet unpublished research on HIV/AIDS and suicide in London shows that in the Riverside district alone the suicide rate among men living with AIDS rose from 4 in 1988 to 96 in 1992. Motivated by his own personal experience ('I have lost too many friends to suicide'), one of the researchers is convinced that many of these AIDS suicides were 'unnecessary' and a 'waste of life'. This is because most carers and counsellors were never open to let the suicide option even be discussed. Hence, the desperate cries for help which lay behind these suicides could never be heard.

Without being privy to all the research statistics, I would guess that most of these male suicides were gay men. I suspect that not all the tension they were struggling with was to do with the prospect of future suffering and death. Probably some of it was an inability to find positive meaning for their lives as gay men. As we have already seen, a positive sense of self-identity and of community and social appreciation not only helps towards a belief in one's self-worth. It also fortifies a person for the struggles to be faced in life and even for a positive approach to the process of dying. In her report for the Health Education Authority, *Suicide Issues in a Cohort of HIV Positive Clinic Attenders*, Dr Lorraine Sherr rejects the myth that 'suiciders choose death over life' and that their suicide 'involves a vision of active embracement of death'. She sees this myth as a stumbling block for positive intervention. A change in focus could allow 'for input which could ameliorate some of the life traumas'. That, in turn, might 'allow for life options to be contemplated and release from the notion of death as the only solution'. On my 'exposure' visit to Uganda I had the privilege of meeting an extraordinary group of women 'living positively with AIDS'. They struck me as a powerful witness to the truth of Dr Sherr's point.

If the Christian Churches could accept a positive appreciation of homosexuality and homosexual relationships, it might help homosexual persons feel that 'it is wonderful for us to be here'. In his remarks about the ethics of suicide, Karl Barth suggests that it is no help to say 'Thou shalt not kill' to a person contemplating suicide. What such a person needs to hear is 'Thou shalt live'. In other words, such a person needs assurance that his or her life is worth living. Such a conviction can be conveyed only through the experience of feeling loved and appreciated as the person one is. That might possibly be what many of these suicides in Riverside could not feel. It is certainly not the feeling that Simon's Christian friends aroused in him. As Christopher O'Hare observed: 'Simon killed himself because he and others thought that he should not be who he was.' Any alleged presentation of the Gospel which gives such a message is not 'good news'. It cannot claim to be Christian. It is not from God.

In contrast to that, the Gospel heard by Nigel Sheldrick, a gay man who died of AIDS in June, 1990, seems more like the authentic Christian Gospel since it was heard clearly by him as life-enhancing 'good news'. That is why, shortly before his death, he was able to give the following personal testimony:

> Of course, there have been hard times. I have gone through a lot of loneliness and despair and anger and grief of all sorts. But I know and have experienced that when I get rid of all the emotional rubbish and my anger, when I am able to shout, 'Oh God, this is awful. I have been abandoned and I am on my own', then fear subsides and faith and hope emerge. For me the opposite of hope is fear and when I have gone through utter despair and lost even hope, it is like entering a new doorway; faith emerges out of my discharging anger and fear and I have sensed a tremendous feeling that everything is all right in the universe. I remember once after a hard workshop I came out of my loneliness and despair and experienced the most inspirational ten days of my life. I felt a sense of connectedness with people and the world. I sensed that life was chaotic but beautiful. I felt like singing and dancing. I felt like going up to people and grabbing them and saying, 'You are wonderful, you really are bloody wonderful.' I wanted to say to them all that your pain and hardships are good; embrace it and experience it and you can change it . . . I feel at the moment that, just possibly, physical death is a doorway to all of us realising that incredible spontaneity and potential that is continually bursting around and in us. Perhaps heaven and hell are sort of within us and we have the potential to life in heaven now – if we can go through the veil of anguish and tears that we have built up over the years. If only we could really see our splendour, if only we could all see each other's splendour what a different world it would be. (Nigel Sheldrick, personal testimony written shortly before his death in January 1990, in James Woodward, ed., *Embracing the Chaos: Theological Responses to AIDS*, London, SPCK, 1991, pp. 20–1)

I found those words very reminiscent of a passage from Thomas Merton's book, *Conjectures of a Guilty Bystander* (London, Sheldon Press, 1977 edn):

> In Louisville . . . in the centre of the shopping district, I was suddenly overwhelmed with the realisation that I loved all those people, that they were mine and I theirs, that we could not be alien to one another even though we were total strangers. It was like waking from a dream of separateness, of spurious self-isolation in a special world, the world of renunciation and supposed holiness. The whole illusion of a separate holy existence is a dream . . . It is a glorious destiny to be a member of the human race . . . If only everybody could realise this! But it cannot be explained. There is no way of telling people that they are all walking around shining like the sun . . .
>
> Then it was as if I suddenly saw the secret beauty of their hearts, the depths of their hearts where neither sin nor desire nor self-knowledge can reach, the core of their reality, the person that each one is in God's eyes. If only they could all see themselves as they really *are*. If only we could see each other that way all the time . . . I suppose the big problem would be that we would fall down and worship each other. (pp. 153–5)

Perhaps the Good News in a 'time of AIDS' is inviting us to fall down and 'worship' gays and lesbians *as the persons they really are in God's eyes!*

5

WHAT THE CHURCHES ARE SAYING

CHURCH STATEMENTS: LISTENING TO AN ONGOING CONVERSATION

Though some writers of Church statements on moral matters might believe that they are producing 'timeless moral guidance', it is probably truer to say that they are joining in a conversation sparked off by contemporary concerns at a particular moment in time. Today, for instance, a whole variety of new developments and possibilities are opening out. In response to this situation the underlying question that needs to be faced by the Churches is: 'How far are these developments humanly transforming or deforming and how can we ensure that this new knowledge and technology is used in a way which will be humanly beneficial?'

Admittedly, some Church leaders may not see their statements as joining in a conversation. They may believe they are ending the conversation by issuing a definitive moral judgement on the issue under discussion. However, people skilled in the art of good conversation are able to cope with that kind of intervention. Consequently, although such statements may be uttered in a definitive tone, they can be interpreted by any skilled conversationalist in the group as being expressions of concern, highlighting issues of importance which the speaker feels might be in danger of being overlooked. Interpreted in this way, even very authoritarian statements can contribute rich insights to the conversation without unduly disrupting its flow.

An image similar to that of conversation is the 'weaving' image which is used by Elizabeth Stuart in her book *Just Good Friends*. This is an image which is particularly attractive to many women. In the following passage Stuart applies the weaving image to theology. This image can also be applied to ethical statements coming from the various Churches. Her comments about theology can help us see the differences between the Churches on sexual ethics in a more positive light:

> I think the metaphors of spinning and weaving are helpful here. We take our own experience, share it, analyse it and spin it into threads of knowledge which can be woven with the threads of others. We cannot know whether a pattern will emerge. If it does, we may claim it as a moment of revelation, a pattern, a map, a trace of the divine . . .
>
> I always think that Christian debate on issues like sexuality might be much more constructive if both sides began every book, every speech, every conversation by acknowledging that they might be wrong. We can only weave what we find, but we might be weaving a false trail – our neighbour may be right. This is why we must always be prepared to listen to our neighbour and why we have a duty to scrutinize our neighbour's tapestry and speak out if we are convinced that it will lead not to a God of justice but down a road of injustice . . .
>
> When we weave our webs of theology we are not weaving shrouds to wrap the dead body of God in, nor are we capturing her, sewing her into the patterns we create. In a very real sense we are weaving the tracks of a God who has already moved on, the trails of a trail-blazer. So all our theology is partial, transitional and at best but a shadow of the truth . . . We also believe that the Spirit has been blowing through history for thousands of years, inspiring the spinning and weaving of tapestries of theology . . . There are undoubtedly many who like to raid their ancestors' store cupboard and hold fast to their tapestries. They prefer a religion dead, a Spirit pinned down like a butterfly. Anything to avoid having to take the risk of spinning and weaving for themselves . . . We are forever the early Church, incarnating the mighty wind or the gentle breath of God, forever running to catch up with it, forever weaving theological meaning out of our experience. (pp. 12–16)

Stuart adds the comment that 'theologians are spinsters and weavers' (p. 16). Perhaps the same could be said of those who try to weave the differing convictions of their Church members into one comprehensive report.

Our reading of Church statements on sexual ethics will also be affected by who we consider to be legitimate participants in the conversation. Some would restrict the conversation to a Church's own members while others would want it to be ecumenical. Many, myself included, would see it as involving everyone in society. There is a hint of this in a sentence in the Church of Scotland's Panel of Doctrine report, *On the Theology of Marriage*, presented to their 1994 General Assembly: 'We affirm that God is God of the whole world, and that understanding of his truth comes in a process of unfinished conversation between the Church and world as we seek to understand the Word of God in Scripture, tradition and current Church practice' (n. 6.6). In the same vein the Vatican II Pastoral Constitution, *The Church in the Modern World (Gaudium et Spes)*, is presented as the Church's contribution to a conversation with the modern world. In this view the Churches are trying to understand the lifestyle of people today so that they can appreciate whatever good there might be in it. Their question, 'What is going on here?', would not be spoken in the tone of an investigating police officer but in an enquiring voice, signalling a desire to understand.

Naturally, determining what are the criteria for discerning what is transforming from what is deforming is bound to be itself part of the conversation. What was said in Chapter Two about social construction is relevant here. The fact that certain concrete ethical norms for sexual behaviour are found in the Bible or in tradition does not automatically provide us with a satisfactory answer to today's problems. The way to show due respect for these norms is not by giving them absolute value and treating them as unchangeable, but by understanding them in their social context so that we can appreciate how they might have served human transformation at that time. Such a critical analysis is not aimed at destroying the old. In fact, it wants to make sure that the enduring richness at the heart of traditional wisdom is not lost in the process of leaving behind patterns of thinking which were considered correct in their day but which have now been superseded by our new knowledge and deeper understanding. This renewal process is very different from the attitude of extreme liberals for whom anything goes as long as it 'feels' right for a person. They also disrupt the conversation since for them there is nothing worthwhile to discuss. Criteria for what is transforming or deforming have gone out of the window, since all that matters is an individual's inner conviction.

In chapter 1 of his book, *Religion and the Making of Society: Essays in Social Theology* (Cambridge University Press, 1994), Charles Davis insists that real conversation is impossible without all the participants agreeing on certain basic ground-rules for the conversation. He suggests two such ground-rules. One is that we can attain truth about reality. So our conversation is worthwhile. We have something to talk about. The second is that we can never attain absolute truth about reality. So I can never absolutize my approximation of the truth and so call a halt to the conversation. This implies that participants in the conversation must be open to pluralism but must not confuse pluralism with relativism.

The conversation I am exploring in this chapter is limited to some twentieth-century statements on issues of sexual ethics emanating from Churches in the UK or North America or from their international central bodies. Hence, it does not claim to be an exhaustive study. It looks at a number of statements which either seem to have had a greater impact or whose content seems more substantial and interesting for our exploration. It is remarkable how many of these statements have suffered the fate of being received but not accepted by their Churches. I have not interpreted that to mean that they lack all authority. In fact, they have been produced by groups of people whom these Churches have judged to be both competent and conscientious and to whom they have felt they could responsibly entrust this important work. Perhaps it could even be argued that, as a general rule, these reports are more likely to represent the belief of those in the Churches who are more theologically literate or who have thought more deeply about their faith and its implications for life in the contemporary world. The non-acceptance of these reports is often the result of a desire to avoid polarization in the Church in the face of an intransigent opposition to any change. As we have seen in the previous chapter, the roots for this opposition can sometimes be found in a more fundamentalist reading of Scripture, allied to an a-historical approach to natural law or the theology of creation.

THE CONVERSATION BEGINS: BIRTH CONTROL – DISAGREEING ABOUT THE RELEVANCE OF THE HUMAN CONTEXT FOR MORAL EVALUATION

Birth control, though a concern for women over the centuries, first came to major prominence on the Churches' agenda early in the twentieth century. This was due to the new possibilities opening out as a result of the increased understanding of human reproductive processes. During the early decades of the century, it was becoming more accepted by all Churches, including the Roman Catholic Church, that the mutual love of the couple was a basic good of marriage and not simply a functional good to serve the procreation and upbringing of the children. This was not seen as diminishing in any way the basic good of procreation which still tended to be referred to as the 'primary' good of marriage.

The conversation began to focus on birth control because many couples were no longer content to leave the size of their families to the chance workings of 'nature'. Now that 'nature' seemed less mysterious, and so less 'divine', they began to take measures to make sure that they did not have more children than they could responsibly cope with. Although primitive, and often very unenlightened and ineffective, forms of birth control had been practised over many centuries, it was only now that people began to understand the processes of procreation much more accurately. The era of more knowledgeable and scientific birth control had dawned. So the question was posed: What do the Christian Churches say about contraception: is it morally acceptable? Two early interventions came from the Anglican Church and both were opposed to it. In 1908 the Lambeth Conference declared:

> The Conference regards with alarm the growing practice of the artificial restriction of the family, and earnestly calls upon all Christian people to discountenance the use of all artificial means of restriction as demoralising to character and hostile to national welfare.

It reiterated its position in 1920 when it issued ' ... an emphatic warning against the use of unnatural means for the avoidance of conception, together with the grave dangers – physical, moral, and religious – thereby incurred, and against the evils with which the extension of each use threatens the race'.

Both these statements assumed that artificial contraception was wrong and concluded from this that it was bound to have deforming effects on individuals and society in general. However, neither statement offered any ethical or theological justification for its position.

By a vote of 193 to 67, with 46 abstaining, the 1930 Lambeth Conference changed its stance on contraception. However, no ethical or theological justification was offered for this change of mind. It seems to have based its position on a respect for the consciences of its members. Hence it was prepared to accept the decisions of those who responsibly chose to use contraception:

> Where there is a clearly felt moral obligation to limit or avoid parenthood, the method must be decided on Christian principles.
> The primary and obvious method is complete abstinence from

intercourse (as far as may be necessary) in a life of discipline and self-control lived in the power of the Holy Spirit. Nevertheless, in those cases where there is such a clearly-felt moral obligation to limit or avoid parenthood, and where there is a morally sound reason for avoiding complete abstinence, the Conference agrees that other methods may be used, provided that this is done in the light of the same Christian principles. The Conference records its strong condemnation of the use of any methods of conception control from motives of selfishness, luxury, or mere convenience. (Quoted in John Noonen, *Contraception: A History of Its Treatment by the Catholic Theologians and Canonists*, Cambridge, MA, Harvard University Press, 1965, p. 409)

Noonen comments that this change of stance came 'after the fact'. Birth control was already widely practised. The 1930 Lambeth statement provoked Pius XI to issue his encyclical *Casti Connubii* (1930). The Pope certainly did not see his intervention as a tentative comment to fellow conversationalists in an ongoing dialogue. His intention was to call a halt to the conversation, since he believed that it was contributing to the moral chaos in the world:

The Catholic church, to whom God has committed the task of teaching and preserving morals and right conduct in their integrity, standing erect amidst this moral devastation, raises her voice in sign of her divine mission to keep the chastity of the marriage contract unsullied by this ugly stain, and through Our mouth proclaims anew: that any use of matrimony whatsoever in the exercise of which the act is deprived, by human interference, of its natural power to procreate life, is an offence against the law of God and of nature, and that those who commit it are guilty of a grave sin. (n. 56)

The encyclical looked at the whole of marriage and examined contemporary threats to it. Within this wider context Pius XI tried to offer ethical and theological grounding for his position. Nevertheless, his interpretation of natural law and his use of the Bible and tradition would hardly be acceptable to Catholic scholars today:

The conjugal act is of its very nature designed for the procreation of offspring; and therefore those who in performing it deliberately deprive it of its natural power and efficacy, act against nature and do something which is shameful and intrinsically immoral.

We cannot wonder than, if we find evidence in the Sacred Scriptures that the Divine Majesty detests this unspeakable crime with the deepest hatred and has sometimes punished it with

death, as St Augustine observes: 'Sexual intercourse even with
a lawful wife is unlawful and shameful if the conception of offspring is prevented. This is what Onan, the son of Juda did, and
on that account God put him to death.' (nn. 54–55)

All these interventions seem afraid of change, even though the 1930
Lambeth statement was prepared to register and respect the
experiential decisions of those practising birth control. Perhaps both
Churches were resisting any change because they could not envisage
how they could alter their teaching on birth control without shaking the
theological foundations of a Christian approach to marriage and sexual
ethics. It was still too early in the conversation for anyone to suggest that
such a shaking of the foundations might not be a bad thing. It might
even provoke a courageous and committed theological investigation
which could renew and enrich our whole theology of sexuality and
marriage. However, that would have meant widening the agenda far
beyond the question of artificial birth control.

The setting up of the Papal Birth Control commission by Pope John
XXIII in 1963 was the Roman Catholic Church's first tentative move
towards this kind of theological investigation. However, the Anglican
Church had already moved a few years earlier. The report *The Family
in Contemporary Society*, commissioned by the Archbishop of Canterbury
in preparation for the 1958 Lambeth Conference, stated that 'there are
very strong moral–theological grounds for regarding the responsible
use of contraception by married persons as morally right' (p. 147).
In its Appendix 1 (n. 8, pp. 120–54) it elaborates for the first time
a substantial theological argumentation for a positive approach to
contraception. It offers a three-pronged line of argument.

First of all, it gave a wider ethical interpretation of the meaning of
'procreation':

> It would now be generally agreed that procreation implies
> co-operation with God in his creative work – that it is really
> creation on behalf of God. It would also be agreed that such
> co-operation in the divine work of creation involves the education
> of the child to maturity, and not merely its begetting and birth.
> Consequently the procreative task of parenthood is not completed
> until the last child is fully adult. To this task, the parent's *coitus*
> makes a valuable contribution. Once conception has occurred,
> it plays an important part in the maintenance of harmonious
> relationship between the couple, and thus promotes the well-being
> of the child, first before birth, and then during the whole period
> . . . of growth towards maturity. (p. 139)

Secondly, it argued that the meaning of any particular act of inter-course within marriage is not self-contained but is bound up with the total pattern of relationship – 'Each act of *coitus* between husband and wife must be seen as part of a total pattern of relationship . . . The morally good act of *coitus* is really that which forms part of a pattern of relational acts consistent with the "proper two-fold end" of sexual intercourse in marriage' (p. 141).

Thirdly, it tackled the issue of 'nature' and argued that, while a couple do not have unlimited dominion over 'nature', they do have the right and responsibility to 'modify and adjust' the natural cycles of fertility and infertility in the interests of their relationship and the wider needs of the community:

> The fact that man in his freedom stands above nature, and is therefore at liberty to interpret sex in terms of personality and relation and to use it for the achievement of personal and relational ends, leads to the conclusion that contraception is morally right in certain circumstances. Thus man may legitim-ately extend the range of non-generative *coitus* as it exists in nature, by the use of contraceptive devices, but only so long as this is done in obedience to relational or social needs. In other words, contraception must always represent a responsible use of human freedom in the interests of personal relationship or of the community. The relational needs of man and woman in marriage may demand that *coitus* shall be independent of natural cycles of fertility and infertility; yet man's liberty of spirit allows him only to modify and adjust, and not to abolish the natural unities of physical sexuality . . . *Coitus* is only 'natural', or consonant with man's true nature, when it exhibits all the characteristics of a responsible personal act expressive of a certain integral relation-ship between the man and woman concerned. (pp. 145–6)

It will be noticed that this three-pronged line of argumentation remains within the traditional theology of marriage. It is committed to 'the proper "two-fold end" of sexual intercourse in marriage' (p. 141). It accepts that we cannot 'abolish the natural unities of physical sexuality' and seems implicitly to identify these with the relational and procreational ends. Hence, it states that 'contraception must always represent a responsible use of human freedom in the interests of personal relationship or of the community'. By situating the individual acts of coitus within 'the total pattern of relationship' and by extending the meaning of 'procreation' to include nurturing and education, this line of theological reasoning is able to argue that even *physically* contraceptive acts can be *humanly* (and so, *morally*) truly procreational and life-giving.

In 1961 the Methodist Conference adopted a similar position in the Addenda they attached to their 1939 Conference statement, *The Christian View of Marriage and the Family*. Provided the means of birth control are mutually acceptable to husband and wife and cause no physical or emotional harm, they see 'no moral distinction' between the practice of continence, the use of the infertile periods and artificial methods of contraception. In support of their position they argue that:

> In the biblical revelation the relational and the procreative functions of sex are equally rooted in the creative purpose of God, and neither is subordinated to the other . . . It is important to recognise that continence may frustrate the relational ends of marriage. Contraception, on the other hand, can assist both the relational and the procreative ends of marriage by promoting marital harmony and enabling parents to space their children. (p. 77)

In 1966 the Papal Birth Control commission arrived at a conclusion similar to that of the Anglican Communion and the Methodist Conference. Although its report was never officially published, the text was leaked to *The National Catholic Reporter* in the United States and was also printed in *The Tablet* and in Peter Harris *et al.*, *On Human Life: An Examination of 'Humanae Vitae'* (London, Burns & Oates, 1968), pp. 216–44. Despite its ponderous language, the following passage, drawn from the accompanying explanatory paper by the sixteen theologians involved in the final report, shows a marked similarity with the theological position presented in the Anglican report. It is commenting on the Vatican II statement that responsible parenthood must be conformed to 'objective criteria' which safeguard both the procreational and relational meanings of marriage 'in the context of true love' (*The Church in the Modern World*, n. 51):

> (a) *The meaning of sexuality in marriage.* 'The responsible procreative community' is always ordered towards procreation; this is the objective and authentic meaning of sexuality and of those things which refer to sexuality (affectivity, unity, the ability to educate). So we can speak of the 'procreative end' as the essential end of sexuality and of conjugal life.
>
> But this procreative end does not have to be realised by a fertile act when, for instance, parents already have children to educate or they are not prepared to have a child. *This obligation of conscience*

for not generating springs from the rights of the already existing child or the rights of a future child. *A child has a right* to a 'community of life and unity' so that it can be formed and educated. Therefore the procreative end is substantially and really preserved even when here and now a fertile act is excluded; for infecundity is ordered to a new life well and humanly possessed. Man is the administrator of life and consequently of his fecundity.

(b) *The meaning of mutual giving.* On the other hand, sexuality is not ordered only to procreation. Sacred Scripture says not only 'increase and multiply' but 'they shall be two in one flesh,' and it shows the partner as another helpful self. In some cases intercourse can be required as a manifestation of self-giving love, directed to the good of the other person or of the community, while at the same time a new life cannot be received. This is neither egocentricity nor hedonism but a legitimate communication of persons through gestures proper to beings composed of body and soul with sexual powers. Here intervention is a material privation since love in this case cannot be fertile; but it receives its moral specification from the other finality, which is good in itself, and from the fertility of the whole conjugal life. (Harris *et al.*, *On Human Life*, p. 213)

This line of thought is also found in the 'Theological Report' section where we read:

The morality of sexual acts between married people takes its meaning first of all and specifically from the ordering of their actions in a fruitful married life, that is one which is practised with responsible, generous and prudent parenthood. It does not then depend upon the direct fecundity of each and every particular act. Moreover the morality of every act depends upon the requirements of mutual love in all its aspects. (p. 232)

This conclusion and the line of argument supporting it were not accepted by the Pope. In 1968 Paul VI issued his encyclical letter, *Humanae Vitae*. Although its first half laid great emphasis on the personal dimension of marriage and the importance of the couple's loving relationship, the Pope insisted on 'the inseparable connection, established by God, which man on his own initiative may not break, between the unitive significance and the procreative significance which are both inherent to the marriage act' (n. 12). Although he claims to be arguing from 'laws written into the actual nature of man and woman' (n. 12), in fact, his focus seems to be more on the nature of the sexual act itself rather than on the nature of the human person.

Consequently, he insists that interference with nature at this level is outside human dominion: 'Just as man does not have unlimited dominion over his body in general, so also, and with more particular reason, he has no such dominion over his specifically sexual faculties, for these are concerned by their very nature with the generation of life of which God is the source' (n. 13).

Clearly this intervention breaks the natural flow of the conversation. It seems to be going back over old ground and disagrees with the interventions of the other three interlocutors mentioned above. Though its tone is less autocratic than that adopted by Pius XI in *Casti Connubii*, it still sees itself as a definitive ruling which should bring the discussion to a close. However, a number of Roman Catholic Bishops' Conferences from different parts of the world soon join in the conversation. None of them express outright disagreement with the Pope. That would break the internal conversational rules usually observed by bishops within the Roman Catholic community. However, quite a number of them inform the members of their local Churches that, if, after serious study and reflection, they find they cannot accept what the Pope has said, they should not look upon themselves as second-class Catholics because of that. In other words, they are implicitly toning down the definitive tone of the Pope's letter. This is very helpful to the other participants in the conversation.

Something similar has happened more recently. Pope John Paul II has spoken out against contraception in even stronger language than Paul VI. However, the impact of his utterances has been softened by various semi-official interventions. A very striking example is the 1994 ARCIC II Agreed Statement, *Life in Christ: Morals, Communion and the Church*, a statement which is still under consideration by the relevant authorities in both Churches. This statement examines the disagreements between the two Churches on certain particular moral issues, including contraception. It sums up the disagreement very clearly:

> The disagreement may be summed up as follows. Anglicans understand the good of procreation to be a norm governing the married relationship as a whole. Roman Catholic teaching, on the other hand, requires that each and every act of intercourse should be 'open to procreation' (n. 80)

The commission are quick to perceive that the real point at issue would seem to be 'the moral integrity of the act of marital intercourse' (n. 81). Both traditions accept that this moral integrity means that the husband and wife hold together the two basic goods of marriage, that is, their loving relationship and the procreation of children. They go on to state: 'For Anglicans, it is sufficient that this respect should characterise the married relationship as a whole; whereas for Roman Catholics it must characterise each act of sexual intercourse' (n. 81). What is most interesting for the ongoing conversation, however, is the next paragraph which reads:

> The Roman Catholic doctrine is not simply an authoritative statement of the nature of the integrity of the marital act. The whole teaching on human love and sexuality, continued and developed *in Humanae Vitae*, must be taken into account when considering the Roman Catholic position on this issue. The definition of integrity is founded upon a number of considerations: a way of understanding human persons; the meaning of marital love; the unique dignity of an act which can engender new life; the relationship between human fruitfulness and divine creativity; the special vocation of the married couple; and the requirements of the virtue of marital chastity. (n. 82)

If the paragraph ended at that point it would be tantamount to saying that the Roman Catholic position has much deeper foundations than the Anglican position and that is why they are different. However, the paragraph goes on to state:

> Anglicans accept all of these considerations as relevant to determining the integrity of the marital relationship and act. Thus they share the same spectrum of moral and theological considerations. However, they do not accept the arguments Roman Catholics derive from them, nor the conclusions they draw from them regarding the morality of contraception.

If I interpret the commission correctly, the import of this paragraph would seem to be as follows. The Roman Catholic position has tended to be presented by authority as a matter of major importance since it is bound up with some fundamental truths drawn from the theology of marriage and sexuality. In other words, the Roman Catholic intervention is saying: 'We cannot accept contraception because, if we do, all these other basic truths are threatened.' The Anglican reply is: 'But we are able to accept contraception and we do not find this puts at risk the fundamental truths of the theology of marriage and sexuality which we hold to just as firmly as you do.'

The two Churches are saying more than that they agree to differ. The Catholics, for instance, are not saying to the Anglicans: 'You say you accept these basic truths about marriage, but I know you don't really. If you did, you would not come to the practical conclusion you do.' Quite the contrary. Both sides are actually agreeing to accept the integrity of their two positions. This means that the Roman Catholic participants are implicitly recognizing that these basic truths are not necessarily bound up with a rejection of contraception. Put more simply, the issue of contraception is not the major issue the Catholic Church tends to claim it is. This seems to be implied even in the opening section of the statement:

> The widespread assumption . . . that differences of teaching on certain particular moral issues signify an irreconcilable divergence of understanding, and therefore present an insurmountable obstacle to shared witness, needs to be countered. Even on those particular issues where disagreement exists, Anglicans and Roman Catholics, we shall argue, share a common perspective and acknowledge the same underlying values. (n. 1)

The disagreement between the two Churches on the issue of contraception provides an interesting example of disagreement between Churches on a particular moral issue. The fact that such disagreement exists can affect how we receive a particular piece of teaching in our own Church. I drew attention to that in an article on the moral teaching of the 1992 *Catechism of the Catholic Church*:

> Since Vatican II, any presentation of Catholic faith must have an ecumenical dimension to it. This entails more than a longing for the unity for which Christ prayed. It also involves a recognition that God's Spirit is at work in other Christian churches. It is in this spirit that the moral section of the Catechism needs to be read. This implies that, when there are particular issues of moral disagreement between the major Christian churches, the Catechism's presentation of the current authoritative Catholic teaching should not be presumed to be the final and definitive Christian position on this topic. The Catechism offers a helpful ecumenical service in presenting the authoritative Catholic position. However, it would ecumenically harmful if such a presentation was understood to carry such authority that any other position must be rejected as unchristian. ('The Catechism and moral teaching: 10 tentative tips for readers', in *The Month*, July 1994, p. 267)

WIDENING THE AGENDA OF THE CONVERSATION: GIVING MORE IMPORTANCE TO RELATIONSHIP – A QUAKER VIEW OF SEX

All the above statements see the procreation and education of children and the faithful love of their parents as equally important – and inseparable, at least within the overall context of a marriage. They also recognize that marriage alone provides the setting needed to attain these two basic goods of sexual loving.

However, in practice the scene has been changing. The co-equal status of these two goods is no longer being taken for granted – and so their inseparability is being questioned. The experience of a loving sexual relationship is assuming more importance in the eyes of the young – and even the not so young. The couple's relationship is seen to be important in its own right and not just for the sake of the children. Couples marry because they love each other and not just because they want children. Awkward questions such as the following begin to be raised once the focus changes from the procreational to the relational and a loving relationship is seen as a good thing in its own right, quite apart from providing a loving context for the upbringing of children:

1. What about a marriage where there has never been such a loving relationship or where it has ceased to be loving and has, in fact, become destructive and deforming? Is any Christian witness given by staying faithful to such a relationship? If not, and if the couple divorce, is any Christian witness given by refusing the possibility of a new loving relationship, if such an opportunity presents itself?

2. If a loving relationship is so important, would it not seem to need as much testing before final commitment as does religious life, for instance? Could not living together before marriage be better described as 'living in responsibility' rather than as 'living in sin'?

3. What is so sacred about a formal marriage ceremony? If cohabiting couples enjoy a truly loving and committed relationship, are they not being faithful to the heart of what Christians believe about sexuality and love?

4. What about such a loving relationship between two homosexual persons, especially if it is granted that their homosexual orientation is natural for them and if experience seems to show that a faithful homosexual loving relationship can be a grace-filled transforming experience?

5. Is it possible to sustain only one such loving relationship? Or does such a loving relationship also include the possibility of lesser loving relationships which do not threaten the major relationship?

6. What about loving relationships in the lives of people who choose to live single or celibate lives? Are deep loving relationships for such people possible and even desirable? Or are they incompatible with their chosen lifestyle?

The first 'Church' statement to acknowledge, and even welcome, this kind of challenge to traditional sexual ethics was *Towards a Quaker View of Sex*, published by the Society of Friends in 1963. It is headed 'An essay by a group of Friends', thus indicating that its views 'do not necessarily reflect the attitude of . . . the Religious Society of Friends'.

This document caused a furore when it first appeared. Its lasting significance is indicated by the fact that it is still in print today over thirty years since its publication. It began with an open acknowledgement of the changing lifestyle of contemporary society. The tone of this acknowledgement is not one of decrying the modern age but simply registering it and even acknowledging that many of those involved would seem to be people of integrity. Its authors write:

> These appear to be the developments we are faced with today:
> a. A great increase in adolescent and pre-marital sexual intimacy. It is fairly common in both young men and women with high standards of general conduct and integrity to have one or two love affairs, involving intercourse, before they find the person they will ultimately marry.
> b. It is even more common for those who intend to marry to have sexual intercourse before the ceremony. This is true, probably, of a very large number of young people in all classes of society, including often those who have a deep sense of responsibility.
> c. The incidence of extra-marital intercourse is great, but it is not possible to estimate whether there is an increase. There must be very many instances which do not lead to divorce or obvious harm and which are kept secret.
> d. A wider recognition, and probably acceptance, of the 'homosexual way of life', and a greater awareness of sexual deviations of all kinds. (p. 8)

The authors believe that sexuality is a fact of nature, powerful but in itself morally neutral. As Christians they rejoice in it as a gift of God, though they recognize that it can be misused (p. 12). They locate the basic moral criterion for judging whether sexual behaviour is transforming or deforming in the quality of the relationship and not in the physical nature of the act of intercourse (p. 41). They suggest that three qualities characteristic of Quakers might add something distinctive to their contribution to the ongoing conversation about sexual ethics: (1) their belief in the equality of men and women; (2) how they see the ongoing conversation; (3) their refusal to make any distinction between the sacred and the secular and so, as a consequence, their recognition of the intrinsic sacredness of the sexual relationship itself:

> There are certain historical characteristics of the Society of Friends that ought specially to lead us to a clear and wholesome understanding of the significance of the sex relationship. The Society has upheld throughout the three hundred years of its history the personal and spiritual equality of the sexes. It has an attitude to authority that enables it to say in the words of John Robinson's farewell to pilgrims setting off for the New World in 1620: 'The Lord has yet more light and truth to show forth' – and on every conceivable question. For Friends, God's will for man can never be circumscribed by any statement, however inspired; the last word has never yet been spoken on the implications of Christianity, and every religious expression is open to critical examination. Quakerism involves a continuous search; and, because it is a genuine and not a formal search, it may lead to surprises and unexpected demands. Lastly, Quakerism has never accepted a distinction between the sacred and the secular . . . In sexual matters the unity of the sacred and the secular involves this implication: that the sacramental quality of a sexual relationship depends upon the spirit and intention of the persons concerned, not upon any atmosphere or circumstance provided from outside. (pp. 10–11)

Chapter IV of the report carries the title 'A New Morality Needed'. The new morality they are looking for is one which recognizes the primacy of love over external rules of conduct:

> Nothing that has come to light in the course of our studies has altered the conviction that came to us when we began to examine the actual experiences of people – the conviction that love cannot be confined to a pattern. The waywardness of love is part of its nature and this is both its glory and its tragedy. If love did not tend to leap every barrier, if it could be tamed, it would not be the tremendous creative power we know it to be and want it to be. (p. 45)

Nevertheless, the authors are aware that such an emphasis on the primacy of love could easily be interpreted as a *carte blanche* for an 'anything goes' approach to morality. This could be interpreted as implying that private judgement reigns supreme, that the responsibilities of marriage and family mean nothing and that sin no longer features as a possibility in the sphere of sexual behaviour. They make it quite clear that they reject all of these implications:

> Although we cannot produce a ready-made external morality to replace the conventional code, there are some things about which we can be definite. *The first is that there must be a morality of some sort to govern sexual relationships.* An experience so profound in its effect upon people and upon the community cannot be left wholly to private judgement. It will never be right for two people to say to each other 'We'll do what we want, and what happens between us is nobody else's business.' However private an act, it is never without its impact on society, and we must never behave as though society – which includes our other friends – did not exist. *Secondly, the need to preserve marriage and family life has been in the forefront of our minds throughout our work.* It is in marriage that sexual impulses have their greatest opportunity for joyful and creative expression, and where two people can enter into each other's lives and hearts most intimately. Here the greatest freedom can be experienced – the freedom conferred by an unreserved commitment to each other, by loving and fearless friendship, and by openness to the world. In marriage, two people thus committed can bring children into the world, provide them with the security of love and home and in this way fulfil their sexual nature. *Finally, we accept the definition of sin given by an Anglican broadcaster, as covering those actions that involve exploitation of the other person.* This is a concept of wrong-doing that applies within marriage as well as outside it. It condemns as fundamentally immoral every sexual action that is not, as far as is humanly ascertainable, the result of a mutual decision. It condemns seduction and even persuasion, and every instance of coitus which, by reason of disparity of age or intelligence or emotional condition, cannot be a matter of mutual responsibility. (p. 46, italics in text)

Though written over thirty years ago, this essay by a group of Friends still makes very challenging reading. As a contribution to the ongoing conversation, reactions to it varied from outright condemnation to qualified support. The 1966 report *Sex and Morality*, by a British Council of Churches (BCC) Working Party, followed the Quaker agenda to the extent that it paid more attention to the possibility of an approach to sexual ethics which placed less emphasis on hard and fast rules and left more room for personal moral judgements in specific situations. Perhaps the report which accepted most fully its 'quality of relationship' criterion was the report of another BCC Working Party published fifteen years later, *God's Yes to Sexuality* (Rachel Moss, ed., London, Collins, 1981).

None of these reports deny the goodness of marriage. In fact, the Quaker report is very lavish in its praise of the marriage relationship. However, they insist that it is the quality of the relationship which is the ultimate norm. In fact, the final sentence of the later BCC report makes explicit something which is only implicit in the Quaker report. That is that even the marriage relationship itself is to be judged according to the 'quality of relationship' criterion. 'We have rejected the idea that marriage is the normative pattern of relationship against which all other possibilities are to be measured' (p. 172). Once this point is made in the conversation, it is natural that attention is directed towards those marriages where the relationship has broken down and the relationship has begun to take on a destructive quality.

MARRIAGE BREAKDOWN: A CHURCH OF ENGLAND CONTRIBUTION

Because of the importance now being given to the human relationship, the issue of marriage breakdown began to occupy the attention of the Churches. Couples were getting divorced because they found that their relationship had broken down and was proving mutually destructive. There was a move to change the divorce laws in the United Kingdom since they seemed to be adding to the negative impact of marriage breakdown on couples and their children.

In 1966 the Church of England joined in the debate with the report of a group set up by the Archbishop of Canterbury, *Putting Asunder: A Divorce Law for a Contemporary Society*. The first of a series of major reports on marriage and divorce from the Church of England, it made an important contribution to civil divorce law in the UK by its advocating that the main ground for divorce should be moved from matrimonial offence to irretrievable breakdown of the marriage. The main concern of most of the subsequent Church of England reports was whether, in the light of the apparently clear prohibition of divorce by Jesus, divorcees could be remarried in church. In exploring this question, the 1972 report by the Church of England Commission on Christian Doctrine of Marriage, *Marriage, Divorce and the Church*, tried to balance the 'relationship' and 'institution' dimensions of marriage.

Of even greater importance was the 1978 report *Marriage and the Church's Task* from the Church of England Marriage Commission. It accepted that the commitment given in marriage is 'unconditional'. Consequently, it saw 'the task facing the Church' as being one of fashioning 'a discipline which holds before those who are married, and those about to marry, the challenge of unconditional love, while offering to those who have failed in their marriage the possibility of a new beginning' (n. 266). Crucial to this report is what is meant by the marriage bond. The commission sees different dimensions to this bond and states that it is the 'personal bond' based on 'mutual love' which weaves together all these various strands (n. 95). The commission is even prepared to acknowledge an 'ontological character' to this personal bond:

> The marriage bond unites two flesh-blood-and-spirit persons. It makes them the persons that they are. It binds them together, not in any casual or peripheral fashion, but at the very centre of their being. They become the persons they are through their relationship to each other. Each might say to the other: 'I am I and I am you; together you and I are we'. Since the marriage bond is in this way a bond of personal *being*, it is appropriate to speak of it as having an 'ontological' character. (n. 96)

While the commission rejoiced that 'there actually occur such ontological unions between man and wife, unions which, as a matter of fact, nothing can dissolve' (n. 97), they tried to face the problem of relationships which had broken down. Only one member of the seventeen-person commission interpreted the notion of 'ontological' bond as meaning that it 'was impervious to time and change, participating in the eternity of being' and so 'once made, could not be unmade' (n. 98). The rest of the commission saw this unbreakable union as something which the couple were committing themselves to bring about rather than as a reality in existence from the moment they entered marriage:

> the bond which was established by consent and commitment was not to be identified outright with the ontological bond which united two persons at the centre of their being and which, in its perfectness, was in fact unbreakable. This latter bond was not simply a bond of commitment grounded in promise and obligation. It was a relational bond of personal love, a compound

of commitment, experience and response, in which the commitment clothed itself in the flesh and blood of a living union. The commitment looked forward to this deeper union of love. Indeed, in faith it anticipated and proclaimed it. Nevertheless, *this deeper union had still to be realised* . . . In one sense, the commitment made, the marriage already existed. But in another sense, the making of the marriage was a continuing process. The bond of commitment had to realise itself as a bond of love. (n. 99)

The commission were not prepared to accept marriage breakdown simply as a fact of life with no ethical relevance. They recognized that something deforming had happened. Without necessarily imputing personal guilt to the couple themselves, they acknowledged that 'human failure and sin' are part of the picture in the tragedy of marriage breakdown:

> There is something radically wrong when a marriage does break down. Marriages *ought* to be indissoluble! However, most of us reject the doctrine that marriages *cannot* by definition be dissolved. It is only too possible for men and women in particular cases to break the bond which God, in principle and in general, wills to be unbreakable, and to put asunder what God, in his original purpose, has joined together. Therein lies the measure of human failure and sin. (n. 100)

The latest report from the Church of England on this topic, *An Honourable Estate*, 1988, looked at the problem of how far clergy are obliged to celebrate the marriages of all who ask, regardless of their understanding of marriage.

A ROMAN CATHOLIC CONTRIBUTION – VATICAN II

An important Roman Catholic contribution to the conversation was made by the bishops assembled for the Second Vatican Council. The Pastoral Constitution, *The Church in the Modern World (Gaudium et Spes)*, promulgated in 1965, marked a major development in the Roman Catholic Church's approach to sexuality and marriage. The relevant paragraphs (nn. 47–52) need a fuller commentary than is possible here to bring out their richness and carefully nuanced meaning. Perhaps the main developments found in them could be summed up in the following eight points:

1. They adopt a new vocabulary for speaking about marriage,

preferring to speak of marriage in terms of covenant or relationship rather than in the language of contract (n. 48);

2. They drop the use of the terminology of 'primary and secondary ends of marriage'; preferring a more 'personalist' approach to marriage, even defining marriage as a relationship in which the couple 'mutually bestow and accept each other' (n. 48);

3. Faithful married love has its source in God's love and when expressed in 'mutual self-bestowal' is 'caught up into divine love' (n. 48). By implication, therefore, the expression and deepening of this love by sexual intercourse is also 'caught up into divine love', something which many Christian writers down through the centuries would have found difficult to accept!;

4. The life-long character of marriage is based principally on the nature of the couple's loving relationship rather than on the needs of children (n. 48);

5. Children are the 'supreme gift' of the love relationship rather than the primary end of marriage (n. 50);

6. Limiting the size of their families can be a responsible (even, at times, necessary) decision for Christian couples (n. 51);

7. Not being able to express their love sexually for each other can be harmful to a couple's marriage: 'Where the intimacy of married life is broken off, it is not rare for its faithfulness to be imperiled and its quality of fruitfulness ruined' (n. 51);

8. There is nothing wrong in a married couple making love even when their intention is not to have children, since that maintains 'the faithful exercise of love and the full intimacy of their lives'. The actual 'means' of birth regulation adopted are to be judged ethically not simply in the light of the couple's intention but according to 'objective criteria' based on 'the nature of the person and the person's acts' (n. 51).

THE JOY OF MARRIED SEXUAL LOVE: A METHODIST CONTRIBUTION

The God-given goodness of the sexual expression of human love (cf. n. 3 above) is taken a stage further in the 1980 Methodist report, *A Christian Understanding of Human Sexuality*. As we saw in the previous chapter, due to disagreement over its use of Scripture in its treatment of homosexuality, this report was sent back to the circuits for further discussion. The ongoing conversation between the Churches is enriched by this report's recognition that the joy of sexual love is God-given and something to be celebrated. A married couple's mutual sharing in this joy is a vehicle for their expressing deep feelings of love, forgiveness, support, and self-giving which help to build and affirm their personal relationship:

> Sexual love, including genital acts when they express that love, shares in the divine act of loving with every human activity which is creative, dedicated and generous. Yet until recently Western Christian attitudes have shown little enthusiasm for the idea of sexual love as an element of Christian living . . . (A28) Despite the biblical references to the joy which God gives to his children, most Western traditional Christian attitudes have not accepted enjoyment as an essential part of God's design for mankind. Physical pleasures have been frequently equated with sin. Since sexuality provides some of the greatest pleasures, it has therefore been most suspect. This rejection of joy warps the Christian understanding of the love of God, the goodness of his creation and the wholeness of human nature . . . Sexuality is not merely useful. It is enjoyable, purposeful and fulfilling. It is a means whereby man and woman may glorify God and grow in the fulfilment of one another. (A29)

> Every physical expression of love from the most tentative to the most complete brings new dimensions to the loving relationship. A glance, a touch, an embrace, a kiss, increasing physical intimacy and genital encounter – the value of each lies in the quality of meaning and emotional response which it conveys together with the appropriateness of the action to the fundamental relationship of love in terms of the commitment of the persons in any given situation. (A36)

> When it is the appropriate expression of love and mutual discovery, coitus is the physical enjoyment of a present union and a symbolic anticipation of that fuller union with the other which belongs to the kingdom of heaven . . . The passion and ecstasy which may accompany true love-making – especially in genital encounter – are to be seen as total self-giving and not regarded as simply a loss of control. (A38)

Largely thanks to the work of Dr Jack Dominian, the truth of the above position is now widely accepted even within the Roman Catholic Church.

A later Methodist document, *Report of Commission on Human Sexuality*, presented to Conference in 1990, goes still further in celebrating the goodness of sexual joy in the love-making of a married couple. It recognizes that 'the context for sexual intercourse is much wider than the strength of the former link with procreation suggested' since its purpose is to 'form, develop, reinforce and renew a bond of love within the context of a committed, personal, loving relationship, and to give and receive mutual pleasure in one another'. It links this insight to the advent of effective contraception:

> In recent years, advances in contraception have helped hetero-sexuals to celebrate sexuality and to engage in sexual activity for itself and not only for its procreative purpose. It is this separation of sexual intercourse from procreation which has brought about a freedom, known already to lesbians and gay men, to value sexual activity for itself . . . This separation has invited heterosexuals to ask the question: if a sexual act is not for procreation only, what else is it for? The answer for all of us is that this act is but one expression of our sexuality, and that our very sexuality belongs integrally to our being human. Sexuality is essential to our humanity. (nn. 14–15)

TWO CONTRIBUTIONS ABOUT HOMOSEXUAL RELATIONSHIPS

To accept, as the above statement does, that sexual loving does not need to be justified by any procreational purpose but that it is good 'as an expression of unity between two persons . . . within the context of a committed, personal, loving relationship' leads the conversation to look at another question. Should it not follow from this that sexual love in a 'committed, personal, loving homosexual relationship' should also be regarded as good? In Chapter Four we have already listened to what the Methodist and Roman Catholic Churches have said on this issue. Here we will listen to contributions from two other Churches. Though this might seem to be giving inordinate attention to the issue of homosexuality, we would be missing out on some of the richness of the conversation if we overlooked them. The first speaks about the theology of creation in a very challenging way and the second gives a very helpful summary of alternative Christian positions.

1. The Church of England

The Church of England looked at homosexuality in two of its reports. Although *Homosexual Relationships* (1979) is in some ways the more substantial of the two, *Issues in Human Sexuality* (1991), from the House of Bishops, makes a more interesting and provocative theological contribution to our on-going conversation. That is the report considered here.

When they consider the issue of homosexuality, the bishops set out 'two fundamental principles of equal validity and significance':

> The first is that homophile orientation and its expression in sexual activity do not constitute a parallel and alternative form of human sexuality as complete within the terms of the created order as the heterosexual . . . Heterosexuality and homosexuality are not equally congruous with the observed order of creation or with the insights of revelation as the Church engages with these in the light of her pastoral ministry. (5.2)
>
> (The second is that) homosexual people are in every way as valuable to and as valued by God as heterosexual people. God loves us all alike, and has for each one of us a range of possibilities within his design for the universe. (5.4)

Part of their argument in favour of their first principle lies in their belief that 'the physical order is sacramental':

> If the physical differentiation between the sexes is not only relevant to the biological process of reproduction but is also integral to the personal spiritual realities of mutual self-giving, parenthood and complementarity, then this is a major instance of a principle that lies at the heart of the Christian world-view: that the physical order is sacramental . . . Our bodies can be the means of forwarding a spiritual and, where there is a living relationship with God, a divine purpose in our lives. For this to happen, however, there has to be a harmony between the physical and the spiritual. When we think of our bodies in this light, we see that they need to be used in a way that is both proper to themselves and in harmony with the spiritual realities we are trying to express and foster. Psychologically, this corresponds to the ideal of an integrated human personality, where body, feelings, mind and spirit work fully together. Theologically it corresponds to the desire that every aspect of ourselves should be aligned with God's will. (4.19)

However, the bishops' positive pastoral attitude towards Christians living in a gay or lesbian relationship and expressing their love for each other sexually seems to by-pass this principle altogether. Instead, it is based on respect for the conscientious decisions of such homosexual persons rather than on any possibility that their homosexual orientation and behaviour might have any goodness in itself:

> Of Christian homophiles some are clear that the way they must follow to fulfil this calling is to witness to God's general will for human sexuality by a life of abstinence . . . (5.5)

> At the same time there are others who are conscientiously convinced that this way of abstinence is not the best for them, and that they have more hope of growing in love for God and neighbour with the help of a loving and faithful homophile partnership, in intention lifelong, where mutual self-giving includes the physical expression of their attachment. In responding to this conviction it is important to bear in mind the historic tension between the God-given moral order and the freedom of the moral agent. While insisting that conscience needs to be informed in the light of that order, Christian tradition also contains an emphasis on respect for free conscientious judgement where the individual has seriously weighed the issues involved. The homophile is only one in a range of such cases. While unable, therefore, to commend the way of life just described as in itself as faithful a reflection of God's purposes in creation as the heterophile, we do not reject those who sincerely believe it is God's call to them. (5.6)

The compromise character of this pastoral approach led the bishops to insist that their acceptance of a homophile lifestyle on grounds of conscience did not apply to clergy living in 'sexually active homophile relationships' (5.17).

This report has been criticized for its inconsistency. For instance, Michael Banner, in his article, 'Five Churches in search of sexual ethics: A short commentary on a statement from the House of Bishops and some other recent reports', in *Theology*, 1993, pp. 276–89, remarks that, unlike Paul to the Corinthians, the word from this report 'certainly seems like Yes and No – or rather No and Yes' (p. 276). However, he gives two cheers to the bishops for their treatment of the order of creation, seeing it 'as at the very least indicating a sense of the importance of a theme in Christian ethics which the present era is inclined to forget' (p. 281). As we shall see a little later, he himself is firmly wedded to a Barthian interpretation of the doctrine of creation.

In their ethical evaluation of homosexuality the bishops' position is very similar to the official Roman Catholic position, though their pastoral approach is very different. They insist that a homosexual orientation is contrary to God's order in the world. Hence, in no way is it a gift from God. They are implicitly saying to gay men and lesbian women: 'You are wrong in what you believe about yourselves, but we recognize your sincerity. Since we respect your conscience, erroneous though it is, you may be part of our church fellowship provided you are not part of the ordained ministry.' Theologically, the main argument on which they base their stance seems to be that heterosexuality, understood as 'man–woman complementarity' (4.17), is a fundamental dimension of God-given creation. Hence, for the bishops one of the special difficulties for homosexuals is the fact that 'their sexuality can be a barrier rather than a help toward full man–woman complementarity' (4.19).

2. The Evangelical Lutheran Church in America

The 1993 report *The Church and Human Sexuality* came out of an ongoing discussion of sexuality over four years within the American Lutheran community. It bears the sub-title, 'First Draft of a Social Statement'. This is because the writers found among Church members three different positions, all supported biblically and theologically. Consequently, they judged that their community needed to continue talking and listening to each other on this issue: 'Because of the differences present in our church, we are challenged to listen respectfully to the witness of those whose perspectives differ from our own' (p. 16). This 'first draft' was never voted upon and did not result in any official policy position of the Evangelical Lutheran Church in America. Nevertheless, its very succinct summary of three different stances on gay and lesbian relationships found among Lutherans is worth quoting *in toto* since it reflects the different positions found within most Churches involved in the ongoing conversation:

Among members of our church, three responses are common:

Response 1 To love our neighbour who is homosexual means to love the sinner but to hate the sin. The church should be loving and accepting of persons who are homosexual, welcoming them as members, but clearly oppose their being sexually active. All such activity is contrary to God's Law. Negative moral judgements should be upheld and homosexual persons expected to abstain from sexual activity. Repentance should be expected from those who do not abstain, trusting that out of divine grace God will forgive them, as God does all repentant sinners.

Those who hold this position tend to view homosexuality as a disease or a serious distortion resulting from the Fall. Because of this disease or distortion, such persons cannot responsibly live out their Christian freedom through sexual activity, even in a committed relationship. Some believe that homosexual persons can be changed in their sexual orientation, so that the loving response is to encourage and help them to change. Others believe that a homosexual orientation is basically given, that change is unlikely, and that lifelong abstinence is the only moral option.

Response 2 To love our neighbour means to be compassionate toward gay and lesbian persons and understanding of the dilemma facing those who do not have the gift of celibacy. It is unloving to insist upon lifelong abstinence for all persons whose homosexual orientation is an integrated aspect of who they are. To tell them they will never be able to live out who they are as sexual beings is cruel, not loving. Thus, the loving response is to tolerate, perhaps even support mutually loving, committed gay and lesbian relationships.

Those who hold this position tend to view homosexuality as an imperfection or example of brokenness in God's creation. Although homosexuality may not reflect what God intends for our sexuality, in an imperfect world we must respond realistically to the situations in which people find themselves and promote what will be less harmful to individuals and communities. It is more in keeping with God's intentions to live out one's homosexuality in a loving, committed relationship than through loneliness or casual sexual activity. This is somewhat analogous to how remarriage following divorce is viewed today: as a necessary accommodation in a broken world.

Response 3 To love our neighbour means open affirmation of gay and lesbian persons and their mutually loving, just, committed relationships of fidelity. Such relationships are the context for sexual activity that can be expressive of love for one another. Prohibiting this expression of love is incompatible with the love of God we know through Jesus Christ, who challenged religious rules that hindered love for the neighbour. God's redemptive and sanctifying activity empowers gay and lesbian Christians to live lives of responsible freedom, including through faithful, committed sexual relationships. It is untenable to maintain that those who are gay or lesbian should have to live lives of secrecy, deception, or loneliness, alienated from self, others, and God.

Those holding this position tend to view homosexuality as another expression of what God has created. Homosexuality should be lived out with ethical qualities, boundaries, and structures consistent with those that apply to heterosexual persons. The church should move toward a practice of blessing committed same-sex unions. (pp. 15–16)

THE CHURCH OF ENGLAND AND COHABITATION: INTRODUCING 'DIVERSITY OF LIFESTYLE' AS A NEW TOPIC IN THE CONVERSATION

If the quality of the relationship is the major factor to be considered, the conversation among the Churches could not fail to face up to the issue of cohabitation. What is so sacred about a formal marriage ceremony? If a cohabiting couple are truly living a committed and faithful personal relationship, are they not honouring the heart of what Christians believe about sexuality and love? Clearly, this is not just an abstract debating issue. Young couples in Britain and across Europe seem to be voting with their feet. In a relatively short period of time cohabitation seems to have become an acceptable practice.

In its 1995 report *Something to Celebrate: Valuing Families in Church and Society*, the Church of England was the first to raise cohabitation as an issue in the conversation between the Churches. This report, focusing principally on the family, was written by a Working Party of the Board of Social Responsibility. It soon came under fire in the Synod, including a broadside from the Archbishop of Canterbury, Dr Carey. The objection was that it was undermining the institution of marriage. This seems rather unfair. The foreword, written jointly by the Bishop of Liverpool and the Bishop of Bath and Wells, states clearly that 'the vision of the Report is to affirm marriage as the basic framework' (p. ix). Moreover, the section on cohabitation, which occasioned much of the criticism, reiterates the Report's emphasis on the centrality of marriage:

> The Christian practice of lifelong, monogamous marriage lies at the heart of the Church's understanding of how the love of God is made manifest in the sexual companionship of a man and a woman. The increasing popularity of cohabitation, among Christians and non-Christians, is no reason to modify this belief. On the contrary, it is an opportunity and a challenge to the

> Church to articulate its doctrine of marriage in ways so com-
> pelling, and to engage in a practice of marriage so life-enhancing,
> that the institution of marriage regains its centrality. (p. 118)

For our purpose what is of greatest interest in this report is its
treatment of the diversity of family structures. This is linked to one of
the three main themes of the report highlighted in its Introduction,
namely, diversity and respect. There it insists that 'we cannot assume
that a particular shape of family, to the exclusion of all other, is God-
given', though it is also careful to note that 'diversity, like uniformity,
should not be accepted uncritically' (p. 6). As the Introduction
implicitly notes, this respect for diversity links in with the notion of
learning from experience how God is working in people's lives:

> Welcoming diversity implies a respect for differences. It is
> important to be open to how God is working in people's lives
> as they are . . . There is no value in telling them that they ought
> to start from somewhere other than where they are. (p. 7)

Chapter 4, 'Theological perspectives on families', notes the *de facto*
diversity in family patterns that has existed in the past and continues
to exist today. It suggests that the Church will only grow in wisdom in
this whole area of life through listening to all the ways God is speaking
to us, including the findings of historians and the social sciences:

> Christians celebrate the goodness and providence of God both in
> creation and in the process of history. One dimension of God's
> goodness is clearly to be seen in the rich diversity of creation and
> the variety of ways in which human beings live together in their
> different cultures and societies. This variety of patterns of human
> community exists likewise in those primary communities we call
> 'families'. The cross-cultural researches of anthropologists and
> sociologists and the findings of historians of the family help us to
> appreciate the diversity and to recognise that whatever we affirm
> as being good and true for family life has to take this seriously. This
> has important implications. It suggests that no single form of the
> family is a kind of God-given ideal, in relation to which every
> other form has to be compared and evaluated . . .
>
> What is necessary is to develop and practise ways of living
> together which seek to embody the wisdom which Christians
> believe comes from God and is revealed in Christ and the
> Christian way. This wisdom is deep and wide. It draws on biology
> and what the natural sciences teach us about gender, sexuality,
> reproduction and human development. It draws also upon history

and what the humanities and social sciences have to say about what people past and present have found to be good and life-giving ways to live together and raise children. It draws upon the witness of scripture and tradition to Christ as the wisdom of God who gives life and light to the world. This wisdom is God's gift to humanity. It is for people in nuclear families and people in extended families. It is for people whose families are dispersed. It is for lone-parent families. It is for people in a cohabiting relationship. It is for people in a same-sex relationship. It is God's gift to all humanity in all its diversity. (pp. 87–8)

The authors insist that openness to diversity 'does not mean that "anything goes" in forms of family life' (p. 88). However, as Christians we should not feel threatened by what we experience as different, as though 'our own position is the last barrier against a tidal wave either of moral chaos or of moral oppression' (p. 88). The authors add some wise advice, very relevant in view of the conversation idiom pursued in this chapter: 'our vocation is not to shout at each other from entrenched positions, but to walk alongside each other so that we can share what wisdom we have about the family in a spirit of humanity and love' (p. 88).

Against this background, the authors of the report go on to make some challenging statements. For instance, though they agree with the House of Bishops in *Issues in Human Sexuality* (1991), that 'the greater the degree of personal intimacy, the greater should be the depth of personal commitment' (p. 108), they are still prepared to suggest that there might be room in sexual ethics for a positive appraisal of sexual loving on the part of some mature non-cohabiting single people:

> We are aware of the many mature single people in contemporary society who do not feel called to be celibate and yet seek to live creatively and ethically in right relationships with others, with themselves, and with God. We believe that one of the tasks facing the Church in the years ahead will be to develop a sexual ethic which embraces a dynamic view of sexual development, which acknowledges the profound cultural changes of the last decades and supports people in their search for commitment, faithfulness and constancy. (p. 109)

The report's treatment of cohabitation notes that 'It is expected that by the year 2000, four out of five couples will cohabit before they marry' (p. 209). The Working Party had been asked to pay particular attention to this issue. They make a number of suggestions as to why cohabitation is so much on the increase in Britain and elsewhere and

note a variety of reasons why this development is giving people cause
for concern. At a practical level, the authors offer two pieces of advice
to the Church. The first concerns the phrase 'living in sin':

> The first step the Church should take is to abandon the phrase
> 'living in sin'. This is a most unhelpful way of characterising the
> lives of cohabitees. It has the effect of reducing cohabitation in all
> its complexity of intentions and variety of forms to a single,
> sensationalist category. Theologically and ethically it represents
> a serious failure to treat people as unique human beings. It
> perpetuates the widespread misconception that sex is sinful and
> that sin is only about sex. (p. 117)

The second piece of advice advocates a more open and less judge-
mental approach to cohabitees on the part of Church congregations:

> Anxiety among church goers about cohabitation is best allayed,
> not by judgemental attitudes about 'fornication' and 'living in sin',
> but by the confident celebration of marriage and the affirmation
> and support of what in cohabiting relationships corresponds most
> with the Christian ideal. Being disapproving and hostile towards
> people who cohabit leads only to alienation and a breakdown
> in communication. Instead, congregations should welcome
> cohabitees, listen to them, learn from them and co-operate with
> them so that all may discover God's presence in their lives and in
> our own, at the same time as bearing witness to that sharing
> in God's love which is also available within marriage. (p. 118)

By situating them in the general context of its diversity theme, the
report's 3-page discussion of lesbian and gay partnerships, though
short, is very positive. However, it adds nothing of real substance to
what we have heard already in the conversation. One final point of
interest in the report is found in its section on 'Households'. It warms
to the suggestion made in a submission by the Jubilee Policy Group
that 'relational values' is 'a more helpful and more inclusive term'
than 'family values'. Moreover, under the heading of 'essentially
healthy relationship values' it lists: 'trust, fidelity, honesty, truthfulness,
commitment, continuity, compassion, self-sacrifice, forbearance, kind-
ness, generosity, sharing respect, understanding, loyalty, co-operation,
solidarity' (p. 121).

TWO CONTRIBUTIONS DRAWING TOGETHER THE MANY THREADS OF THE CONVERSATION

1. The Church of Scotland

In 1994 the Church of Scotland General Assembly was faced with two different reports dealing with sexuality and marriage and also touching on homosexuality. 'On the theology of marriage' was a report from the Panel on Doctrine. The other report, entitled 'Human sexuality', was from the Board of Social Responsibility. (Texts in *The Church of Scotland: Reports to the General Assembly, 1994*, pp. 257–85; pp. 500–16)

The report commissioned by the Panel on Doctrine was accepted unanimously by the Working Party which prepared it. However, six of the fourteen members of the Panel itself opposed it and insisted on their note of dissent being added to the report. In the light of the issues we have been considering, some of their reasons for dissent are particularly interesting:

4. The Report effectively drains away authority from the Scriptures by diverting the question of what the Bible *means* and *teaches* into an endless and drifting 'conversation'.

6. The Report virtually ignores the doctrine of creation and thus underplays the significance of the male–female distinction as a structure of creation and divine gift and fails to recognise marriage as a God-ordained institution.

7. The Report, in its recommendations concerning same-sex relationships and pre-marital sex, weakens the Church's ability to speak prophetically by implying that these forms of sexual relationships are *morally equivalent* to marriage, thereby weakening the normative status of marriage and diminishing the significance of the two-parent family.

Despite these criticisms from six of the Panel on Doctrine, I found this report to be a very well-informed, up-to-date and responsible piece of writing on the theology of marriage. It opens with a discussion of scriptural interpretation which fully recognizes the role played by social construction and the implications of this for theology:

> It is an insight distinctive to the 20th century that our interpretation of Scripture is likely to be bound up with our cultural and linguistic presuppositions. Access to wide comparative data from a large number of disciplines, the cross-fertilisation of cultural exchange and interaction, the studies in history and social science which document the impact of social conditioning, all

raise general awareness of the way our ideas are embedded in a particular inherited social structure. At a theoretical level, the 'sociology of knowledge' suggests that all human understandings of reality are likely to be relative to the specific cultural context in which people operate. (3.3)

Within the churches, there is increasing recognition that all theology is bound to be 'contextual' – not just in the sense of *addressing* a particular situation, but in the sense of *emerging from* particular patterns of speech, thought and understanding (often unselfconscious) and deeply embedded in structures of social, linguistic or cultural belonging. The idea that there can be an uncontested 'universal theology', free from such cultural conditioning and filtering, seems to many implausible. For those who want to claim absolute certitude and authority in matters of doctrine or ethical perception, such recognition of cultural relativism seems threatening to the claim that God reveals himself. It may, however, be seen not as a loss of religious nerve, but as an affirmation of how partial, or even distorted, the human reception of God's self-disclosure is liable to be; in which case it is seen as proper humility in the face of the variety of ways that God's truth has been understood within different traditions and at different periods of history. 'Where pluralism is denied, finitude is forgotten, and faith is corrupted into an idolatrous absolutising of one of its particular expressions.' (3.4)

After stressing the importance of marriage in a very moving and powerful passage (4.2), the report goes on to speak of marriage in the language of 'sacramental mystery', drawing inspiration from the Orthodox sense of the sacramentality of creation:

Marriage at its best is transparent of the goodness of God, offering glimpses of the joy, fidelity and communion which mark the life of the Kingdom, and enjoying the benediction of God's lovingkindness. This sense of marriage as a sacramental mystery is confirmed by the widespread human experience of the marriage relationship as the most precious and deep exploration people make in their life history. (4.7)

The report also recognizes very realistically the extra strains on the marriage relationship today, including the fact that 'marriage often assumes structures of an earlier patriarchal society which are no longer acceptable to many people' (7.4d). It even acknowledges that the Church has colluded in this situation:

We must recognise that the Church has, in much of its traditional utterance and practice, accepted and reinforced a patriarchal account of family structures which makes women subservient to men. This account has treated women, informally if not officially, as domestic servants or possessions, whose time and energy are at the disposal of husband and family with or without consent. (7.7)

When it considers same-sex relationships, the report notes that some Christian gay and lesbian partners see their relationship as 'God-given and God-sustained' (9.2). The report then makes a very challenging statement which, in fact, is quite consistent with the flow of the conversation as we have seen it developing between the Churches:

> If we wish to suggest that the ultimate vindication of a marriage lies in the free, mutual giving and receiving of selfhood, which makes for the wholeness of the partners, body, mind and soul, there has to be significant reason given for denying a comparable wholeness to people of same-sex orientation. (9.3)

A similar point is made a few paragraphs later:

> Since, for us, marriage is no longer tied to procreation but is vindicated by the love and commitment it sustains, and since we believe God welcomes and invites such relationships between men and women for their own sake, the relevant question is whether he may welcome them also for homosexual people. (9.6)

The report answers that question by stating:

> Given our increasing understanding of human sexuality in this century, it seems arbitrary and cavalier of the heterosexual majority to deny their gay brothers and sisters the fullness of relationship they themselves enjoy – unless they are sure that such relationship is utterly repugnant to God, or damaging to wider human wellbeing. (9.6)

The final conclusion of the report brings the whole discussion back to the basic focus on the quality of relationships, suggesting that marriage at its best offers a God-given paradigm of a loving and life-long relationship but querying whether that paradigm need exclude the goodness of other relationships involving sexual intimacy:

> We believe that the emphasis of our advocacy of marriage must not be about the legitimacy or illegitimacy of specific sexual acts, but about the virtue of cherishing, mutual, communicative, loving relationships. It is these relationships which show what it means that we live, in the image of God, not as self-sufficient units, but

in the giving and receiving of life from one another. Marriage is a God-given paradigm of that life-long exchange of life, and we share the desire to affirm that. What divides us in the Church is whether other relationships involving sexual intimacy may also belong, however imperfectly, to that affirmation of self-giving and receiving mutuality, and may be offered to God in good faith as a response to his gifts of human love and sexuality. (10.9)

The second of the two reports to the General Assembly is entitled *Human Sexuality*, and comes from the Board of Social Responsibility. It concentrates on sexuality in general rather than on marriage. Its main focus is pastoral. Its discussion of homosexuality looks at views about possible causes of the homosexual condition and examines different ways of interpreting the witness of the Bible regarding homosexuality. While the report deliberately refrains from giving its full support to either side of the debate, in the course of its treatment it poses two challenging questions to the Church:

Sexuality lies at the heart of our self-hood and sense of identity, developing with us from the beginning of life. In the light of this, how are those who find themselves attracted to someone of their own sex to express their sexuality in their living and relating? Such fulfilment and realisation will follow many pathways including possibly genital satisfaction. In view of the difficulties inherent in this question, it seems logical to ask to what extent those of the minority orientation of homosexuality are to be free to enjoy God's gift of sexuality. Since sexuality is an essential part of a person's identity, can this be denied without severe psychological and emotional damage? (8.2.1)

It is the quality of the relationship which is paramount and in this context sexuality plays a significant part. Sexuality, therefore, serves primarily to initiate, cement, and enrich relationships. Procreation is a 'second order' function of sexuality, ordained of God but not its main role, which is to do with relationship. It is clear that many human partnerships display valued and sought-for qualities and we must ask whether such relationships, which include the possibility of genital sexuality, are to be denied to those who are of the same sex. (8.4.6.4)

2. The Presbyterian Church (USA)

A very interesting contribution to the conversation is the report of a Special Committee on Human Sexuality presented to the 1991 General Assembly of the Presbyterian Church (USA). It is entitled *Keeping Body and Soul together: Sexuality, Spirituality and Social Justice*. Like some other officially commissioned reports we have looked at, it was received but not endorsed by the General Assembly. In fact, it occasioned a very heated dispute both prior to and within the Assembly.

Michael Banner, in his article referred to earlier in this chapter, is very scathing about this report, dismissing most of it as 'mere rhetoric' ('Five Churches in search of sexual ethics', p. 282). He criticizes it for lacking any appreciation of 'what belongs to the created order and what does not'. This latter criticism reflects Banner's own Barthian standpoint which, as he himself explains, stands four-square behind a male–female interpretation of gender differentiation which he sees to be an essential element in the doctrine of creation:

> To be created in the image of God means for the Book of Genesis, so Barth alleges, to be created male and female, and it is in the creation of woman, with and for the man, that both creation accounts see the completion and perfection of God's work. Furthermore, he argues, we can assert (on the strength not only of the Book of Genesis but also on the basis of the rest of the Old and New Testaments which find such meaning and significance in the man/woman relationship) that it is in the duality of male and female that humankind is determined in its creaturely being as the covenant-partner of God; that is to say, that this earthly determination of humankind as man and woman corresponds to the divine determination of humankind for covenant with God. (p. 282)

It is this which lies behind Banner's criticism of the report as being based on a 'popular and thorough-going individualism'. For him the report 'baulks at the idea that men and women are made for fellowship and thus are, as individuals and alone, in some sense incomplete' (p. 283). In her essay, 'Homophobia, heterosexism, and pastoral practice' (in Jeannine Gramick, ed., *Homosexuality in the Priesthood and the Religious Life*, New York, Crossroad, 1989, pp. 21–35), Rosemary Ruether rejects Barth's position precisely on the grounds that it is based on a theory of human development that is 'truncated' and merely reflects patriarchal social roles:

> This condemnation of homosexuality as incomplete and narcissistic is a basic reinforcement of heterosexism. Its doctrine that only heterosexual sex is 'whole' is actually based on a truncated human development for both men and women in which both must remain 'half' people who need the other 'half' in order to be 'whole'. This truncated personality development reflects patriarchal social roles.

The male and female stereotypes are asymmetrical and reflect the dominance–submission, public–private splits of the patriarchal social order (Barth, 1961, 116–240).

Against this patriarchal social stereotyping, I would claim that all persons, male and female, possess the capacity for psychological wholeness that transcends the masculine–feminine dichotomy. Once this is recognized, the argument for heterosexuality, based on the genders as complementary opposites, collapses. All sexual relations, all love relations, should be the loving of another person who is complexly both similar and different from oneself. Such relationships should help both to grow into their full wholeness. Complementarity, by contrast, creates a pathological interdependency based on each person remaining in a state of deficiency in relation to the other. (pp. 24–5)

The authors of the report begin by outlining the 'massive, deep-seated crisis of sexuality' in contemporary culture:

This crisis shows itself in distorted, often highly negative attitudes, about sex, bodiliness, and intimacy needs. It is also evident in deeply oppressive patterns of sexual abuse and exploitation. At the heart of this crisis are entrenched patterns of unjust and dehumanizing power relations between men and women . . . The crisis of sexuality we are experiencing is, in fact, a massive cultural earthquake, a loosening of the hold of an unjust, patriarchal structure built on dehumanizing assumptions, roles, and relationships. This unjust structure stifles human well-being and stands in contradiction to the gospel mandate to love God and neighbour as self. (*Keeping Body and Soul Together*, p. 3)

They reject the solution offered by 'sexual libertarians' as failing to recognize that human persons are essentially relational and social beings (p. 5). They then shift the conversation in a slightly different direction by insisting that the justice dimension must be at the heart of any sexual ethic (p. 7). Unfortunately, their notion of 'justice-love' is never explained with any precision. This probably explains some of Banner's dissatisfaction. Yet such imprecision does not invalidate what the report is trying to say through its emphasis on 'justice-love'. Perhaps it should prompt other participants in the conversation to try to give it greater precision and clarity. I find it interesting, for instance, that Professor Enda McDonagh commented recently that the 'quality of relationships' criterion might be given more bite if we looked at relationships from a justice angle.

The report tackles head-on the 'complementary' approach to

gender-differentiation, rejecting totally a gender dualism in which 'neither partner functions – sexually or socially – as a fully integrated person, but rather as a fragmented complementary half' (p. 15). It goes on to insist on the need for a thorough-going structural analysis if the Church is to cope with the challenge of structural injustice entrenched in our culture in the three forms of gender and sexual injustice, racism and economic injustice:

> This challenge requires a critique and reconstruction of the dominant sexual code in our culture . . . Understanding this challenge requires shifting to a structural analysis of sexuality and understanding its social construction. Sex and human sexuality are never simply matters of what comes naturally, but rather always culturally encoded. By this code, sex and sexuality are given distinctive shape. To say that human sexuality is socially constructed or coded is to pay attention to how we give social meaning to our sexuality and how those particular meanings shape, to a very great extent, our attitudes and responses . . . It is our conviction that this patriarchal code, not the persons questioning and deviating from it, is what is morally deficient and unjust. Far from being natural, much less divinely decreed, this elaborate social construction of sexuality is built on two false assumptions: gender inequality and male control of women's lives and their bodies. (pp. 15–16)

As mentioned earlier, Banner dismisses much of the report as 'mere rhetoric'. It might be more accurate to say that the report refuses to stand on the side-lines and dispassionately present two sides of the debate without offering any definite conclusion of its own. Its authors are clearly convinced that patriarchy is evil as well as being all-pervasive. They also believe that patriarchy is not a natural phenomenon. It has been constructed by human agency and the only way it can be eliminated is also through human agency. On the other hand, they are convinced that sexual diversity is a natural phenomenon and is not evil. In the light of these beliefs and convictions it is understandable that much of their writing in the report is very impassioned and almost has a campaigning flavour about it. For them, there are major issues of justice involved here. This presents a dual challenge to the Church – first, to put its own house in order and stop colluding with this injustice, and secondly, to become actively involved in the wider movement to right this injustice.

In the overall context of the conversation taking place among the Churches, perhaps a very impassioned intervention like this has an important role to play. For the most part, those actively involved in the conversation tend to be fairly open-minded and well-informed. Their own hesitations may often come from a concern not to alienate the more conservative members of their Church. In their own minds they may actually agree with some, or even most, of the thrust of the Presbyterian report. To hear it voiced so passionately might be a healthy reminder to them that, ultimately, the Church's mission is not to make sure it keeps all its membership on board but to play its part in forwarding the coming of God's Kingdom in the world. It cannot be denied that the Presbyterian report loudly proclaims the urgency of this task.

CONCLUSION

Throughout the conversation between the Churches studied in this chapter, increasingly the main emphasis has been moving towards the *quality* of the relationship. With the acceptance of the relational significance of human sexuality and the acknowledgement that this is not necessarily or essentially bound up with its procreative function, there has been a growing tendency to make 'quality of relationship' the prime criterion in sexual ethics. For instance, in the debate about contraception, it has been argued that individual acts which are biologically contraceptive can be interpreted as *humanly/ethically* procreative in the light of the procreative quality of the whole relationship. Others have gone further and argued that, since sexuality is primarily relational rather than procreative (children being the fruit rather than the *raison d'être* of the relationship), a committed, faithful sexual relationship can be ethically acceptable even without any intention of having children. Provided the couple are open to life and to other people, the quality of such a relationship can be described as creative rather than procreative. A reinterpretation of the 'inseparable connection' mentioned by *Humanae Vitae* seems to be taking place. As sexual persons, created in God's image, it is the inseparable connection between life and love that we must respect, rather than the 'unitive and procreative significance which are both inherent to the marriage act' (*Humanae Vitae*, n. 12). Our loving relationships must be life-giving in a relational and social sense. This naturally introduces the issue of gay and lesbian relationships on to the agenda. Although they have no procreative dimension, same-sex relationships can also be life-giving and creational and can show all the 'relational values' listed at the end of the previous paragraph. Surely, it is argued, their ethical goodness must, therefore, be accepted – and celebrated.

It has also been claimed that this 'quality of relationship' focus throws light on the problem of marriages which have broken down because the relationship took on a destructive quality. Are Christians obliged to stay in a relationship which is destroying them as persons? Pushing the argument still further, does such a catastrophic deterioration of quality, if irremediable, indicate that there is no longer any real marriage there at all, since, in terms of interpersonal love, the relationship has ceased to exist? That, in turn, brings into the conversation the question of remarriage after divorce. If the first marriage, precisely as a loving relationship, is dead, why should not the partners be able to experience the life-giving healing of a new loving relationship, if the opportunity presents itself?

Another aspect of 'quality of relationships' has found its way on to the agenda after a long and hard struggle by women. For the most part, their voices have not been properly represented in the official Church bodies engaging in the conversation. This explains why, except for the 1991 Presbyterian (USA) report, their position has not been given a major hearing in the conversation. The case being argued by these women is that, very widely, the quality of heterosexual relationships has been corrupted by the all-pervading oppressive influence of patriarchal attitudes and structures. Some are also maintaining that to use marriage, as it exists, as the paradigm for a 'good quality relationship' is unacceptable, since the very institution of marriage has been hijacked by patriarchy.

This, in turn, provides part of the explanation for the next item which appeared on the agenda, cohabitation. It is recognized that, in some instances at least, this lifestyle is embraced as a protest against what is seen to be the oppressive quality of the marriage relationship and as an attempt to build a more just style of relationship built on the foundation of equality and mutuality.

In the background of the whole conversation there has been the controversial issue of how far the quality of the relationship legitimates its expression in sexual activity. Once it became clear that every sexual act was not, by its very nature, open to procreation, it became much easier to accept that the principal significance of the human sexual act was relational, rather than procreational. Moreover, when its biological procreative function came more easily under human control and the risk of an unwanted pregnancy decreased, 'sex is fun' became the popular theme of a permissive society. So the conversation had no choice but to discuss the 'recreational' dimension of human sexual activity. This led to a more explicit acceptance of the joy and pleasure of sex as God-given. However, it also helped the conversation to clarify the Christian position and be able to teach that sexual pleasure and joy is short-lived and delusory if it is separated from its primary context within the full relational dimension of human sexuality. Human sexual joy is personal, not just physical. When it is achieved by reducing one's partner to the level of a sex object, it is dehumanizing and wounding for all concerned. However, that having been stated, the question still remained. Is there something about genital sexual activity which makes it inappropriate and even self-defeating outside a committed and faithful relationship? This seems to be as far as the conversation among the Churches has reached.

In this chapter, we have limited ourselves to eavesdropping on the conversation taking place among some Christian Churches through the various statements on sexuality they have produced. We have only listened to some snatches of their conversation. Although these snatches have been important, there have been other bits of the conversation, of perhaps equal or even greater importance, which we have missed out on due to lack of space and the limitations of the topics under consideration. Furthermore, the conversation we have been listening to is only part of a much wider conversation among theologians and others, inside and outside the Christian community. To some extent, we have already listened to a little bit of that wider conversation in the previous two chapters.

In the next chapter, in the light of that wider conversation and taking account of the Church statements we have listened to, I would like to offer some tentative signposts pointing us towards new directions in sexual ethics. Despite their deficiencies due to the limitations of this study and my own personal inadequacy, I hope they might be helpful to the Churches and to Christians struggling to discern the way forward in this daunting but exciting area of human life.

6

TOWARDS A SEXUAL ETHICS IN A TIME OF AIDS

In the light of what we have seen in previous chapters, there would seem to be a number of important directions in which Christian sexual ethics needs to proceed:

- Since it must flow from a belief in the full and equal dignity of women as human persons, it needs to be purified of any patriarchal influences which have stunted its healthy growth.
- Since it must also believe in the full human dignity of gay and lesbian persons, it needs to be freed from an unhistorical approach to the Bible and natural law which has consolidated rather than challenged homophobic attitudes in the church and in society.
- Since it believes that, as human persons, we are created in the image of the Trinitarian God, it needs to do justice to human sexuality as an important dimension of this God-given giftedness.

Though discussion of any specific ethical issues related to HIV/AIDS will be left until Chapter Eight, the AIDS pandemic will serve as a backdrop for the whole of this chapter. That should ensure that we do not lose sight of the urgency of the justice dimension of sexual ethics, particularly as affecting women and also gays and lesbians. Also, being aware of the human and theological implications of social construction we will be better able to handle tradition as a living and continuing process, as well as seeing human cultures, including the sexual mores and gender roles they incorporate, as open to critical analysis with a view to bringing them more in line with human and Gospel values.

It could be argued that the whole of ethics is 'sexual' since our sexuality is an essential dimension of our being human persons and so affects our whole approach to life and all our relationships. However, it could equally be said that the whole of ethics is 'social' or even 'ecological'. Consequently, we need to define more precisely the specific area of human life and relationships which comes within the field of sexual ethics. Unless we do that, our discussion of sexual ethics will become too wide-ranging to be of any practical help.

I would suggest that sexual ethics covers three main areas: (1) personal identity in so far as it is bound up with our biological and psychological make-up and cultural conditioning and the impact of these on gender differentiation and sexual orientation; (2) relationships of intimacy, their language of communication and the social structures which directly affect them; (3) specifically genital activity and its relational, procreational and recreational potentiality.

That could be stated more simply by saying that sexual ethics covers the whole area of

- who I am as a sexual person;
- how I relate to others as a sexual person;
- how I behave as a sexual person.

Obviously, these are not three separate areas. I only discover who I am through the process of relating to other people; and relating to other people is not a purely internal intellectual process. It involves communication by word and gesture. Sexual ethics explores the specifically sexual component of these three areas. As an ethical enterprise its purpose is not merely to offer an accurate description of what actually *is* going on. Rather it is trying to understand what *should* be going on if we are to live in a way which most truly reflects who we are in all our richness as sexual persons.

Clearly, in one short chapter, it is only possible to offer a few pointers towards a renewed sexual ethics. That is why I have included the word 'towards' in the title of this chapter. It is offered as a modest contribution to a task which is ongoing and in which we all have a stake. In the Introduction to this book I made the comment: 'Paradoxically, I suspect that this chapter is the least important one in the book'. I stand by that statement, not because the topic itself is unimportant but because I recognize that there are many women and men far more competent than I am to write on this theme. I will be very happy if the inadequacies of this chapter serve to stimulate them to offer something far more substantial and pastorally helpful.

SOME FOUNDATIONAL BELIEFS FOR A CHRISTIAN SEXUAL ETHICS FOR TODAY

I would like to explore six important articles of belief which I consider should lie at the heart of a transformed Christian sexual ethics for today:

1. Belief in the full and equal dignity of women as human persons as a major touchstone in our age for judging the credibility of the Church's commitment to the dignity of the human person;
2. Belief in human freedom;
3. Belief in friendship, intimacy and love;
4. Belief in the goodness of the human body, sexuality and sensual joy;
5. Belief in the giftedness of human life;
6. Belief in the uniqueness of the human person and respect for personal conscience.

1. THE FULL AND EQUAL DIGNITY OF WOMEN

The more the experience of women has made its voice heard in the field of sexual ethics, the more the focus has moved from a male concern about penetrative sex to the wider context of the sexual relationship. It is to this context that a transformed sexual ethics should devote most of its attention. For women, sexual ethics has generally begun from the wrong starting-point. It has focused too much on sexual intercourse and on trying to define when it was ethically acceptable. For many women, this is not their main concern. Their main concern is the quality of the relationship. In other words, they are looking for a relationship which fully respects them as women and their equal dignity as human persons. If that is lacking, no other compensating qualities can really redeem the situation. Tragically, as things stand, many women feel they have no choice but to settle for less. They see the relationship they are in, unsatisfactory though it may be in many ways, as the best they can hope for at present. However, they know that their experience falls short of the Kingdom values proclaimed by the Gospel.

A Christian sexual ethics must be able to offer a theological critique of the form of marriage which many women are experiencing as oppressive. Hence, it must not have the institution of marriage itself as one of its bedrock foundations immune from any criticism or questioning. It needs to be able to appeal to something more fundamental which will provide it with a more basic criterion for undertaking a critical analysis of the institution of marriage itself.

That more basic criterion is provided by the overarching principle of respect for the human person. This principle which has been canonized by Vatican II seems to be fully accepted by all the other Christian Churches. It even seems to provide common ground with people of other faiths or none. Of course, such a person-centred morality does not involve any rejection of objective morality. Far from it. Vatican II, for instance, is opposed to any kind of purely subjective morality which would claim that the human subject can decide arbitrarily what is right or wrong. We are not free to create our own morality to suit our own convenience. Vatican II insists that morality must be based on 'objective standards' (*The Church in the Modern World*, n. 51). However, its interpretation of 'objective' is completely person-centred. In other words, these 'objective standards' must be drawn from the nature of the human person 'integrally and adequately considered' (cf. my *New Directions in Moral Theology*, pp. 29–30).

In practice, therefore, specific human actions, sexual intercourse, for example, do not have any in-built moral criterion of their own which is distinct from the human person as a whole and which might require behaviour which is contrary to the good of the human person, integrally and adequately considered. Even such a fundamental human institution as marriage does not have any free-standing independent moral criterion of its own. It can only be properly understood and evaluated with reference to that one all-embracing criterion of the good of the human person, integrally and adequately considered. Of course, trying to discern much more explicitly what that means in practice is a crucial question we all have to face. I have attempted a preliminary sketch of one possible way to answer that question in chapter 3 of my book referred to in the previous paragraph.

As we have already seen, at this *kairos*-moment in history, one of the major signs of the times in our age is a growing awareness among women – and men – that the structures of our world over the centuries have been based upon the assumption that women have a lesser dignity as human persons than men and so are naturally subordinate to them. These structures even include the institution of marriage itself and the even more basic institution of heterosexuality. Consequently, the criterion of the dignity of the human person as applied to a critical analysis of both these institutions must look at whether, in their current form, they adequately safeguard and promote the full and equal dignity of women. Anything in both these institutions that fails that criterion must be clearly rejected by sexual ethics. Such a critique would more appropriately be made by women theologians; that is why this section is so brief.

2. HUMAN FREEDOM

Freedom is an essential dimension of our make-up as human persons. We are responsible for ourselves and cannot abdicate that responsibility to others. We are not simply 'objects' to be used functionally for the convenience of others. Our future is not determined by blind fate or the tyrannical power of 'the gods'. At a very fundamental level, to be human means accepting responsibility for what we do and for the kind of person we commit ourselves to become. This remains true, even though our freedom is limited in many ways and we are, all of us, wounded people, victims of sin in some way or other.

Marriage tended to be the main focus of sexual ethics. Hence, freedom was seen as relevant principally only in so far as it had implications for married couples. Moreover, given the fact that marriage was viewed within the 'contract' paradigm, freedom only seemed to assume importance with regard to entry into marriage. A contract was null and void if not consented to freely. Consequently, in the Roman Catholic Church, for instance, a marriage could be declared null, if one of the parties did not consent freely to it. Once past the point of entry, however, the freedom dimension faded more into the background. According to the 1917 Code of Canon Law the couple gave each other 'a perpetual and exclusive right over the body, for acts which are of themselves suitable for the generation of children' (canon 1081, #2). That implied that each had proprietorial rights to the other's body for sexual purposes. In practice, however, this was usually interpreted as meaning that a husband had the right to demand sex from his wife whenever he wanted it. The extreme to which this teaching led can be seen in a matrimonial jurisprudence decision from the Roman Rota which declared that a marriage was considered to be consummated even if the husband had rendered his wife unconscious in order to penetrate her! The text of the decision stated that 'consummation can be had independently of consciousness and free consent of the will' (cf. T. Lincoln Bouscaren and James I. O'Connor, eds, *Canon Law Digest*, Milwaukee, Bruce, 1961 Supplement, on canon 1119). Since the 1993 Code of Canon Law this appalling interpretation is, thankfully, no longer defensible.

In such an approach to marriage there could be no such thing as rape within marriage. A husband was always within his rights and his wife had no right to refuse. This teaching probably had links with the fact that, in earlier centuries, sexual intercourse, though considered sinful because of its necessary association with concupiscence, was judged by theologians to be justified when it was seen as a way of stopping a husband going off to another woman to satisfy his sexual needs. This seems to have been what was meant by the phrase, *remedium concupiscentiae*. This way of looking at the couple's sexual relationship seems to imply that, if the husband did go off to another woman, his wife was to blame since she had failed to satisfy his sexual passion!

In such an understanding of marriage freedom of choice did not loom large. A wife had no such freedom if her husband wanted to demand his right to have sex with her. This was a 'double-standard' morality. One of the principal qualities looked for in a wife was obedience to her husband. However, he was not expected to obey his wife. He was her head. It was his role to exercise authority. Tragically, at a popular level this offered a justification for the appalling practice of 'wife-battering' if this was the only way a husband could make his wife subject to him. At the end of her essay, 'Historical theology and violence against women: unearthing a popular tradition of just battery', in Carol J. Adams and Marrie M. Fortune (eds), *Violence against Women and Children: A Christian Theological Sourcebook* (New York, Continuum, 1995), pp. 242–62, Mary Potter Engel makes the challenging statement:

> We need to open ourselves to the possibility that discoveries of the interconnection of the ideology of gender inequality and the practice of violence against women in the Middle Ages, Renaissance, and Reformation may inform our understanding of patriarchy and our practice toward women in the present . . . As long as we do not unequivocally reject the ideologies of gender inequality, we will perpetuate that tradition, for there will always be at least one just cause for battery of wives: insubordination. (p. 258)

Today's growing emphasis on the 'quality of the relationship' focuses much more on the couple's shared responsibility for the well-being and growth of their partnership. Consequently, a transformed sexual ethic for today would not interpret matrimonial consent in terms of each partner surrendering their personal freedom or giving up their right to free choice. Consent in marriage is not a *surrender* of personal freedom or individual choice. It is actually an *exercise* of personal freedom. It is making a choice. Each partner is effectively saying to the other: 'From now on, whenever I make a choice, you will be part of the equation. And in terms of our shared life and love together, our decisions and choices will be governed by our mutual consent. I am not surrendering my freedom to you nor am I taking over your freedom. But we are agreeing to exercise our freedom together through our mutual consent. I do not believe I have any right to demand sex from you if you are unwilling – and vice versa. However, we are both committing ourselves to be sensitive to each other's needs and to accommodate ourselves as best we can to those needs, even when, on occasion, they do not fully correspond with our own needs at that time.'

Our capacity to make such a life commitment reveals the profundity and wonder of our freedom as human persons. Human freedom is not limited to our capacity to choose between different options. It also includes something much more mind-blowing than that. Human freedom includes the capacity to determine who we are to become and what we are to make of our lives. It means, for instance, that we can grasp hold of ourselves, as it were, and commit ourselves to another person for life. Far from being a surrender of our freedom, such a life-commitment belongs to the highest level on which we can exercise our freedom. Another name for this kind of highest exercise of our freedom is love. This is a favourite theme of Pope John Paul II, as comes over clearly in his encyclical, *Veritatis Splendor*: 'The Crucified Christ reveals the authentic meaning of freedom; he lives it fully in the total gift of himself . . . Freedom is acquired in *love*, that is, in the *gift of self*' (nn. 85 & 87).

To understand freedom in this way enables us to see that the shift from the 'contract' paradigm of marriage to the 'covenant/ relationship' paradigm has moved the marriage commitment up a further notch in the freedom scale. However, this brings with it higher expectations of marriage. That creates a problem. People may now have these higher expectations of marriage but it does not follow automatically that they have the skills necessary to build a marriage relationship on this higher level of personal commitment.

Some people believe that this 'relationship' approach fosters too romantic a view of marriage. Real-life marriage is more down-to-earth and ordinary. There is probably much truth in that observation. Nevertheless, as we saw in the previous chapter, this 'free giving of self to the other' is the understanding of marriage to which most Christian Churches now seem to be committed. They see it as more in keeping with our dignity as human persons made in the image of a relational God. The danger is that this ideal can too easily become a burden on some couples. Having been encouraged to believe in the ideal, they find themselves, for one reason or another, incapable of realizing it in their relationship. And instead of experiencing from the Church understanding and encouragement to pick themselves up and move forward, they discover that their non-attainment of the ideal is seen as disqualifying them from embarking on any further life-giving loving relationship.

The fact that many marriages are breaking down does not necessarily mean that couples do not believe in this higher-level understanding of marriage or that they do not enter marriage with a real desire to make a go of it. It is more likely either that they have not reached the level of personal maturity needed to undertake such a fundamental commitment or that they do not have the interpersonal skills needed to build a marriage relationship of this kind. They have these high expectations regarding the quality of their marriage relationship but they often discover that the reality of such a high-quality relationship seems to be beyond them.

This might partially explain the increasing popularity of cohabitation. It could well be that many couples, believing that it is the quality of the relationship which matters most in a sexual partnership, want to make sure they get this right. Hence, they move in with each other and start living together without any Church or civil marriage ceremony. They believe that the only way they will find out whether they are capable of such a deep relationship with each other is by trying to live it out in practice. Some may even be put off marriage by the fact that it takes too much for granted. It assumes that from day one they are capable of such a high quality relationship with each other. Even though they would love that to be true, they know they cannot take it for granted. So they settle for a lower level of relationship, one they feel more able to cope with. If it grows into something much deeper, they might be prepared at a later date to celebrate it as a marriage. But for the present, they prefer to leave their options open and wait and see.

It could be argued that what is so tragic is that many of these couples, though saying they believe in freedom, do not really believe in their own inner freedom to be able to make a life-commitment of themselves to each other at such depth. It is as though they do not trust themselves enough to make such a commitment. However, they may be being realistic if, in fact, they lack the personal maturity needed for a life-commitment of this kind. Whether cohabitation encourages the growth of personal maturity is open to question. It would be helpful if there was some experimental evidence available as to whether in practice cohabitation provides a setting which is conducive to such people's growth in maturity.

Without freedom we cannot make moral decisions or act morally. However, freedom is not the only morally relevant factor to be considered. Although good sex, in the full sense of the word, needs to be free, there is far more to good sex than freedom. The catch-phrases, 'pro-choice', 'a woman's right to choose' and 'consenting adults' are all appealing to a very important dimension of ourselves as human persons. That is why they are so attractive. However, they are misleading if they mean that all other considerations pale into insignificance in comparison with an individual's freedom of choice. That is tantamount to an extreme form of liberalism which ultimately is inimical to the true freedom of the human person integrally and adequately considered.

Does the freedom dimension we have been considering throw any light on gay and lesbian sexual relationships? I would offer the following comments:

(a) For most people – and almost universally for men – it seems that the sexual orientation we find ourselves with as we emerge from the turbulence of early adolescence is a given, whatever the causal factors which have brought it about. Being true to that given means accepting it as specifying the sexual giftedness of our lives. However, for some women at least, there seems to be more fluidity about the sexual giftedness they receive as their 'given'. If that is the case, in their living out of that sexual giftedness the basic moral principle guiding them must still be the dignity of the human person. And in fact, respect for the human person seems to lie behind the choice made by many women who 'choose' a lesbian lifestyle. Some are in the process of recovering from a marriage which, for one reason or another, has been experienced as oppressive of their freedom; others are making a 'political' rejection of what they see to be a patriarchal construction of the institution of marriage; others, like Alison Webster, are choosing a lesbian relationship because they deem it to be 'qualitatively superior . . . in terms of mutuality, equality, intimacy, communication and sexual pleasure' (*Found Wanting: Women, Christianity and Sexuality*, London, Cassell, 1995, p. 27). In such cases their choice for the lesbian option could be interpreted as an exercise of their human freedom in line with their respect for the dignity of the human person. That being so, it could be argued that, in principle, their choice is acceptable on moral grounds.

(b) Leaving aside the above-mentioned exceptional case of women who freely choose to follow a lesbian lifestyle, a sexual ethics which encourages gays or lesbians to enter into a heterosexual marriage would seem to be running contrary to a proper understanding of human freedom. It would be asking the impossible of them. Moreover, it would be making this demand in an area which touches the human person at a most profound level since it is where a person exercises his or her freedom in its highest form. Such a request is almost sacrilegious since it fails to respect the inner sanctum of a person's self-identity. Given the relational interpretation of marriage accepted by the Christian Churches today, the only person with whom a gay man or lesbian woman could have such a 'free total giving of self' relationship will surely be another gay man or lesbian woman.

(c) It is claimed that relationships between gay men or lesbian women are no less capable of expressing a 'free total giving of self to another' than heterosexual relationships. If this is true, it means that homosexual relationships can fully respect the 'freedom' criterion for a high-quality human relationship. Hence, unless their relationships could be shown to be 'anti-person' on other grounds, to deny gays and lesbians in the name of morality the possibility of choosing to commit themselves to such a relationship would itself seem to be immoral since it would be denying them the freedom to be themselves at a most profound level of their being. To say that they can still freely choose lifelong celibacy would seem to be playing with words. It is implicitly saying that they *must* choose celibacy and thereby denying them the freedom to choose a faithful gay or lesbian relationship. It would be presenting celibacy as a burden rather than as a gift.

3. FRIENDSHIP, INTIMACY AND LOVE

Our sexuality is an important ingredient of our being relational persons. Although it can be the source of great joy and pleasure for us, the fulfilment of that joy does not lie in self-pleasuring but in the mutual enjoyment of relational intimacy as human persons. André Guindon stresses the fact that 'tradition has never acknowledged as Christian a sexual ethics which construes sexual activity as mere self-enjoyment'. This is not a result of the Church's being wedded to any particular philosophical stance. Rather Guindon insists that a central tenet of

Christian faith lies behind this understanding of our human sexuality. It is ultimately based on 'faith in a triune God':

> Each person does not appropriate the divinity for some sort of self-enjoyment, but refers it totally to the others, the Father begetting the Son, the Son saying the Father, the Father and the Son spiring the Spirit, who is entirely referred to the Father and to the Son in love. On the model of the divine persons in which they believe, human persons receive their identity only by relating to the other. From the days when she took a stand against pagan sexual hedonism, notably through the African fathers of the third century, right up to her indictment of the solipsistic tendency of the contemporary 'sexual revolution', the church, in spite of occasional, clumsy formulations, has never ceased to invite women and men to adopt sexual attitudes and practices which do not enclose them within their own pleasure. Nothing less is at stake than the confession of the triune God. ('Theologian offers Vatican-requested explanations', in *Origins*, 25 February 1993, p. 631)

For Guindon, openness to the other is at the heart of an authentic human self-understanding. It is through encountering the 'other' that, ultimately, the door is opened to our encountering God.

However, this openness to the other applies to the whole of human life. The question we need to consider here is in what way our human sexuality has a special bearing on our openness to the other. On the more general level, the dynamism of our human sexuality acts like a kind of magnet drawing us out of ourselves to others and attracting others to us, whether this is in the heterosexual or same-sex magnetic field. It has something to do with our connectedness as human persons. This glorious gift which we share with the animals provides the precious raw material out of which human beings fashion personal relationships, some of them more explicitly sexual than others. The deeper our personal relationships become, the more intimate is our sharing of ourselves in them. This is what the exchange of a loving friendship is all about, two persons opening themselves out to each other in an atmosphere of mutual trust. Elizabeth Stuart, in her thought-provoking and beautifully written book, *Just Good Friends: Towards a Lesbian and Gay Theology of Relationships*, even goes so far as to offer friendship as a paradigm for human relationships in general and, in particular, for relationships of a more intimate sexual nature. Moreover, she insists that all human relationships are essentially 'embodied' and even extends this to our relationship to the material world:

We are called to relate to the world in friendship: a relationship which as it grows between people results in mutual and equal acceptance, respect and delight, it is an embodied relationship with social and political repercussions. In other words, we are called to delight in the world around us, to approach it in a positive rather than negative manner . . . Our delight in our own embodiment should give us a 'shiver of solidarity' with all other bodies and a desire to work to ensure that all bodies are treated justly: all bodies are well fed, have access to good health care, are well sheltered and so on; and that the body upon which all depend, the body of the earth, is also treated justly. (pp. 213–14)

In some cases, the power of sexual attraction between two people is initially the main, or even the only, thing which draws them together. This can be the prelude to growth into a deep friendship, though that is not always the case. If it never gets beyond the level of sexual attraction, it is a very impoverished version of the quality of relationships two human persons are capable of enjoying. If, in such an instance, the couple's sexual attraction leads to sexual intercourse, there may have been a meeting of two sexual bodies, but only minimally of two sexual persons.

Our sexuality enables us to share a very special kind of intimacy with another person – not just physical intimacy, but a more fully integrated personal intimacy. That profound intimacy can be celebrated, communicated, shared and enjoyed in a very unique way through the highly symbolic physical act of sexual intercourse. Sex is at the service of intimacy, not vice versa. In itself, sex can be experienced as something trivial. Personal intimacy can never be trivial. It is something which engages us at a very deep level of our being.

Of course, not all intimate relationships involve specifically sexual activity. Most people enjoy a number of intimate relationships which are not sexual in the strict sense of the word. Relationships of parents with their children or between siblings are an obvious case in point; but even beyond the family circle most people enjoy intimate friendships of a non-sexual character. A more holistic understanding of ourselves as sexual persons is leading to a recognition that such intimate friendships can be a very healthy part of a celibate lifestyle too.

Many ethical writers today believe that what makes a specifically sexual relationship so special is its depth of intimacy. Consequently, for them the key question is: what precisely has sexuality to do with intimacy and what kind of intimacy should there be for sexual activity, including sexual intercourse, to be appropriate?

They are clear that intimacy is not just about sexual satisfaction. That point is made very strongly by Elaine Storkey:

> Intimacy is not primarily about sexual satisfaction. It can be there in a great variety of relationships, between friends, between those in the same family, as well as between lovers. Intimacy is the sharing of closeness and warmth in a context of vulnerability and openness. It is the trust that, here there is safety, here I will not be betrayed. It is the desire for mutual enrichment, through listening, responding, caring, forgiving, growing. In short, it is the experience of love in relationship with another. It is demanding and time-consuming and requires a solid bedrock of commitment. ('Sex that's only skin deep', in the *Guardian*, 21 October 1995)

Intimacy lies at the heart of sexual ethics. If we are to appreciate human sexual behaviour precisely as human – in other words, as the appropriate behaviour of human persons integrally and adequately considered – we need to see it in the wider context of our profound need as human persons for intimacy. Sexual behaviour only finds its true human meaning in the context of interpersonal intimacy.

This longing for intimacy belongs to the very heart of our being human persons. Despite contrary appearances at times and despite the various ways this deep longing can be wounded in us, we all long to be loved and we only discover our true selves in this experience of loving and being loved. The relational dimension of being human touches the very core of what it means to be a human person. As Storkey insists, it engages the level of our personal being at the point where we are most profoundly fashioned in the image of God:

> Made in the image of God, we need closeness with others in order to express and experience our personhood. And the God who calls us into being, the God who is relationship and love, also calls us into community. In community we are simultaneously taken out of ourselves and fully become ourselves. For we are and always will be persons-in-relationship . . . (*The Search for Intimacy*, London, Hodder & Stoughton, 1995, p. 231)

Storkey maintains that the dominant cultural values of today present an obstacle to the achievement of intimacy. Intimacy can only thrive in a climate of trust since it involves self-disclosure and vulnerability. It entails the risk of opening ourselves to an 'other' with whom we are prepared to share our inner selves, accepting each other's woundedness and, in the process, struggling together towards healing and greater wholeness. Intimacy is based on a belief that it is not good to be alone. In fact, it is not human to be alone.

In contrast to this, the contemporary climate exalts individualism. We will only survive in the human rat-race if we beat our competitors. Self-sufficiency is the key attribute to be fostered. Paradoxically, although we have never been so conscious of the global linkages in human living, we view this global picture merely as an extension of the competitive playing-field. It makes us more aware of who our competitors are and how we can make strategic alliances to conquer them. The context is global, but the driving-force remains self-interest. In the end, it is a matter of the survival of the fittest. As Storkey points out, this public world works out of an ethos diametrically opposed to the ethos of intimacy.

Some may argue that intimacy is fine in its place – and its place is restricted to the field of interpersonal relationships. However, it is unacceptable to make such a dichotomy between so-called 'public life' and 'private life' when we are dealing with human morality. If the overriding criterion is the good of the human person integrally and adequately considered, that criterion demands respect for human persons in public life as much as in private life. To give the last word to economic values is tantamount to rejecting that criterion. Both the social and the relational dimensions permeate the whole of our lives as human persons. If the public climate is one in which individualism is in the very air we breathe, that is bound to have an influence on the way we approach our personal relationships. Schizophrenia is a pathological state – it cannot be accepted as an essential dimension of being a human person. We cannot live our public and private lives out of two contradictory philosophies.

Consequently, it is only to be expected that in our current climate a truly human sexual ethic will be, to a large extent, counter-cultural. It will be an ethic which swims against the tide of those forms of sexual mores which are deeply influenced by contemporary individualism. One such form, for instance, is a very individualist recreational interpretation of sexuality which views sexual activity as a kind of competitive sport in which the whole object of the game is to gain maximum satisfaction for the individuals engaged in it. As with all competitive sports, it accepts that there will be losers. They will just have to grin and bear it. Perhaps they will win next time round!

However, the picture is not one of unrelieved doom and gloom. If, deep in our being as human persons, there is this profound longing for intimacy, it is only to be expected that this will still continue to make its presence felt even in the most hostile climate. Storkey maintains that it is still alive and well. In some ways the prospects look even more promising today than in previous ages. One indication of this is the fact that most Christian Churches now recognize the key importance of the intimacy context for sexual ethics. While not denying the link between human sexuality and the continuation of our human family, they are recognizing that the relational dimension is profoundly tied up with our being made in the image of a relational God.

This is almost turning the earlier tradition on its head. For many centuries, the mainstream of Christian tradition regarded the joys of sexual intimacy as dragging human persons down to the level of brute animals. In other words, they 'brutalized' men and women. Today, on the contrary, the joys of sexual intimacy, when shared in the appropriate context, are seen as 'divinizing' the human persons involved. Though these two positions might seem to be in total contradiction, paradoxically the connecting link which provides a certain continuity between them is the notion of intimacy. Intimacy was always seen to hold the key to what it meant to be human. Augustine brings that out in his much-quoted dictum: 'We are made for you, O God, and our hearts are restless until they rest in you.' Augustine was suspicious of sexual activity because he saw it as an obstacle to this sublime human experience of intimacy with God. Nevertheless, *The Search for Intimacy* would have been a very appropriate title for a book by Augustine since it captures his own thinking so succinctly. However, the contents of such a book as written by Augustine would not include a treatment of how the expression of sexual intimacy is sublimely human and revelatory of God. Augustine's appreciation of what was involved in being human was limited by an understanding of human sexuality which was the accepted wisdom of his day and for many succeeding centuries. Today our more holistic understanding enables us to appreciate that we can experience God not just in the dizzy heights of mystical experience but also in the sublime ecstasy of sexual intercourse within a truly loving and faith-filled intimate relationship.

This longing for intimacy could well be the underlying drive behind the great upsurge in sexual activity today, especially among young people. It is hardly doing justice to what is happening to describe it as an abandonment of morality or an indication of total sexual licence. In company with Elaine Storkey, I believe that the longing for intimacy in people is just as alive as it ever was. However, today people are having to cope with an experience of profound alienation and even meaninglessness. This is partly the fruit of the current ethos of individualism and of a reductionism which assesses everything and everyone purely on their monetary value. People, especially the young, feel alienated – from themselves and from each other. As a result, they want to lose themselves in togetherness. Sadly, many do this by blowing their minds on drugs and communal raves. Many, too, seek an escape from their loneliness in sexual encounters of different sorts.

The tragedy is that they are not finding what they are looking for. This is because they are searching for intimacy in the wrong place. Those who follow the sexual path are looking for it in sexual experience itself, divorced from a truly human intimate relationship which is the only context in which it can really be found. Sexual enjoyment will not quench their longing for intimacy. Real satisfaction will only be found in the intimate joy of mutually shared love. However, this is a much bigger undertaking than a one-night stand or even a much longer transitional and uncommitted relationship. Dr Jack Dominian has repeatedly made this same point in his various writings.

Since this undertaking engages two persons at a very deep level of their humanity, it needs to respect certain basic ground-rules if it is to do justice to the human personhood of the two individuals involved. Much of Storkey's book explores these basic ground-rules for fashioning an intimate relationship. They all revolve around such fundamental issues as trust, self-disclosure, communication, confidentiality, commitment, and so forth. Her treatment of friendship (pp. 151–8) is particularly helpful in this regard.

As Storkey notes, along with many other writers, the search for intimacy seems more in tune with women's natural inclinations than with men's. Women seem to sense its importance in a relationship more easily than men. It stands higher on the priorities of most women. In making this observation, she is not suggesting that intimacy is not a human need, common to both men and women. It is just that women seem more aware of this and more naturally endowed with the human skills needed to fashion intimacy. If this is true, it could be argued that we are living in an age in which the emphasis is moving from a predominantly masculine to a more feminine interpretation of human sexuality.

4. THE GOODNESS OF THE HUMAN BODY, SEXUALITY AND SENSUAL JOY

Such a positive affirmation of the goodness of the body, of our sexuality and of sexual pleasure is in complete contrast to so much dualist thinking which, as we have seen earlier, coloured the earlier Christian approach to sexuality in one way or another. No longer is the passionate and affective character of our sexuality seen as a malign force dragging us down to the level of brute animals. It is now seen as an integral element of our being human persons. We are empowered to raise the sexual giftedness which we share so closely with the animal kingdom to an even higher level through our specific giftedness as humans. This is not a matter of leaving behind what links us to the animal kingdom, rather like a space probe casting off a booster rocket. It is much more a matter of integration. We accept the sexuality we share with other animals and ennoble it still further by stamping it with the specific imprint of our humanity. We are not human despite our being bodily sexual beings. We are human through our being bodily sexual beings. To disown the bodily sexual dimension of ourselves would be to dehumanize ourselves.

There has been an increased emphasis in recent years on the bodily dimension of our sexuality. Among the many books read in the course of my research for this book, four of them carried body-centred titles. They are all important books in their own right: James B. Nelson, *Embodiment: An Approach to Sexuality and Christian Theology* (London, SPCK, 1978); Gareth Moore, *The Body in Context: Sex and Catholicism* (London, SCM, 1992); Peter Brown, *The Body and Society: Men, Women and Sexual Renunciation in Early Christianity* (London, Faber & Faber, 1988) and Elisabeth Moltmann-Wendel, *I Am My Body: New Ways of Embodiment* (London, SCM, 1994). Moreover, James Keenan points to extensive contemporary Christian writing on the theme of the body in his excellent survey article, 'Christian perspectives on the human body', in *Theological Studies*, 1994, pp. 330–46.

In their different ways these writers are all reminding us that our modern emphasis on personal relationship in sexual ethics must not lead us to overlook the important truth that our relationships are mediated through our bodies. Obviously, they are not suggesting that our bodies are simply highly sophisticated communications systems. That would imply that we are persons living inside our bodies and using our bodies to communicate with other persons, a kind of sexual version of e-mail! Bodily mediation goes much deeper than that. As the title of Moltmann-Wendel's book reminds us, we are our bodies. Hence, we do not communicate by means of our bodies. Rather we communicate as body-persons. Consequently, in a specifically sexual relationship a couple are not exchanging love notes through their bodies. What they are doing is loving sexually – and sexual loving can be the medium for expressing a whole rich variety of human feelings and emotions. Moore is making a similar point when he insists that sexual gestures are not merely substitutes for words: 'If Andrew says to Jane: "I love you" and then makes love to her, he is not guilty of repeating himself' (*The Body in Context*, p. 106).

Moore points out that the Catholic Church has consistently condemned sex 'for mere pleasure'. However, he argues that this condemnation has often been misunderstood – even by those proclaiming it. Some have understood it as condemning any direct enjoyment of sexual pleasure, others as forbidding a couple to have sex together for the sake of their mutual enjoyment. Both are a misinterpretation. 'Mere pleasure' was intended to mean depersonalized pleasure separated from any relational significance. Admittedly, many writers interpreted the intensity of sexual pleasure as almost necessarily causing such a separation. Hence, they tended to refer to it as 'lust'. Today our deeper understanding of ourselves as sexual persons leads us to a very different interpretation of sexual loving. An extended quotation from Moore might help to bring this out:

> in any normal sexual activity nobody is out of control. They know what is happening, what they are doing and what they are likely to do; they decide to do some things rather than others; and so on. They may get excited, they may let themselves go, but when they do that they do not in general get out of control. I am not denying that it is possible to lose control of ourselves in sexual activity, to get carried away and do things we would not normally do and of which we may later be ashamed or for which we might reproach ourselves. But when we do that, it is not a matter of the body escaping from the control of the mind . . . It is simply we lose control of ourselves . . .

> . . . neither is it true that sexual pleasure is so great that when it is at its height one cannot think . . . Sexual pleasure is often intense, and it belongs to the notion of intense enjoyment that you are fully engrossed in what you intensely enjoy; you do not want to tear yourself away from it, are not easily distracted, and maybe want more of it. We would only 'be able' to think (i.e. want to think) at the climax if the pleasure were less intense. This

applies not only to sex but to all pleasures which may be intense, such as listening to music. (p. 49)

Moore also quotes a very interesting passage from Aquinas in this connection:

> The abundance of pleasure which is in a sexual act ordered in accordance with right reason is not contrary to the mean of virtue . . . Neither, if the reason cannot freely think of spiritual things at the same time as that pleasure, does that show that that act is contrary to virtue. For it is not contrary to reason if the act of thinking is sometimes interrupted by something which is done in accordance with reason; otherwise it would be contrary to reason for somebody to give himself up to sleep. (*Summa Theologica*, 2–2.153.2 ad 2 – quoted in *The Body in Context*, p. 50)

Theologians in the past, being exclusively male, have tended to focus almost exclusively on the male experience of sexual pleasure. That is beginning to change. In *Sexuality and the Sacred: Sources for Theological Reflection* (London, Mowbray, 1994), a collection of articles edited by James B. Nelson and Sandra P. Longfellow, there is a profound theological reflection on the female orgasm written by Mary D. Pellauer, entitled 'The moral significance of female orgasm: towards sexual ethics that celebrates women's sexuality' (pp. 149–68). The following passage from her article, which is profoundly rich theologically, could never have been written by a male theologian:

> Concentrating, focusing – these are 'mental' abilities that are as much a part of sex as any purely physical abilities. Being fully present, where is the language for this? Meditation is the closest analogue I know; this comparison is surprisingly apt, for both are disciplines of being here-and-now, of letting go . . . (p. 155)

> Orgasm is sui generis. It is paradoxical. Ecstasy is what is at stake here. *Ek-stasis*, standing outside the self, is the closest word for this state. At the same time, it is the most definite incarnation I know outside of childbirth, for in it I am most completely bound to the stimulation of my body. Thus, immanence and transcendence meet here, another paradox . . . It is a limit-experience . . . (pp. 156–7)

> The Western tradition has been quick to talk about the need for spirit or mind to rule the body with its imperious passions. We have been less apt to talk at length about the gifts the body gives to the spirit . . . (p. 161)

A good sexual experience is a source of worth and value to the participant(s). To touch and be touched in ways that produce sweet delights affirms, magnifies, intensifies, and redoubles the deep value of our existence. Ecstasy spills over onto the world outside the bed, not accidentally but intriniscally. It awakens rejoicing, but more: wonder and reverence, the poignant astonishment that we are here, that we live, that anything at all is here, that life can enfold such bursting joy. What if more of life were like this? In my experience, female orgasm is so rich, so abundant in meaning that it is supersaturated with it. It is superabundant, a treasure trove. Women wondering, women marvelling . . . (p. 162)

Sadly, the above description would not be true of every woman's experience of sexual intercourse. Not infrequently, as came out in a survey conducted some years ago by a French Catholic periodical, it is better summed up in the word 'nightmare'. That is tragic and only emphasizes the need for a profound change of thinking and practice in the field of sexual ethics.

A few years ago I was involved in a day for Catholic couples who were all involved in running marriage preparation courses in their parishes. In one session I asked them to think of one thing about marriage which they had never heard mentioned in the pulpit but which they would like to hear said very explicitly. The suggestion which elicited the strongest support was: 'Sex is enjoyable and good'. Christians today are able to see that this statement does not involve a rejection of our earlier tradition. It simply recognizes that when we bring to this tradition the new knowledge and understanding of human sexuality available to us now, the goodness of sexual joy in its appropriate human context is the only conclusion which does justice to the heart of that tradition. Consequently, the message that 'sex is enjoyable and good' is something which the Christian Churches should now be saying loud and clear.

A sexual ethics based on the good of the human person integrally and adequately considered will recognize that to be truly human, bodily sexual pleasure must be personal. In fact, it must be interpersonal. This is because it is the bodies of human persons that are involved. Moore makes this point well:

This flesh cannot be alive without being human flesh, and it cannot be alive without being the flesh of this particular person. To regard Jane as live flesh and without being concerned with her as human being, as person, is not a way of being concerned with her but a failure to be concerned with her. This is what is meant by the Christian insistence that what is important in sexual relationships is that they should be relationships between people. (*The Body in Context*, p. 58)

This is why in prostitution it is the dignity of the prostitute as a human person which is violated by her male client. The word 'prostitution' is misleading since it seems to imply that it is something in which the woman is the main actor. In reality, what occurs is sexual abuse of the woman by her male client since normally he is using his economic power to purchase human flesh without any relationship with the person involved. Moore writes:

> Why, in Christian ethics, cannot sex properly be a transaction, like buying a packet of cigarettes? . . . Because, though I can want a person's body without wanting him or her, I cannot get this body without getting him or her. A human being is his or her body. I cannot get the flesh without getting the person. A sexual relationship, precisely because it is an engagement with a human body, is an engagement with a human being. (p. 60)

Jack Dominian is continually insisting on this point. In his book *Proposals for a New Sexual Ethic* (London, Darton, Longman & Todd, 1977), he writes:

> The evil of our age is not sexual permissiveness so much as the trivialisation of human encounter which, in the name of freedom, encourages the minimum engagement with the maximum haste and the maximum disengagement . . . The trivialisation of our age is not that of sex but of persons, who, in the name of rights and freedom, are sanctifying the partial, the transient, the incomplete, the shallow and who ultimately place each other constantly on the sacrificial altar of the disposable. The evil of our day is disposable relationships . . . (pp. 69–70)

The Church's mistrust of sexual pleasure probably helps to explain why it saw procreation as the primary purpose of sexual intercourse – and of marriage itself. Today a 'relationship' interpretation of the meaning of marriage has changed our whole focus. Relationship is about the shared joy of being together, of sharing all that goes to make up life together. Fundamentally, it is the relationship itself which is pleasurable. Obviously, the pleasure of such a relationship embraces far more than the physical sexual pleasures involved in love-making. Nevertheless, these physical sexual pleasures are an important part of the whole picture. They are a very significant dimension of a couple's shared enjoyment of each other – part of the pleasure of being together and doing things together. Consequently, the bodily sexual pleasure a couple share is something much deeper than the physical sensations of sexual arousal and orgasm. After all, these physical sensations can be experienced even in situations which are far from pleasurable, as in the horror of rape or sexual abuse.

A fairly prevalent attitude to sex today is summed up in the phrase, 'sex is fun'. Many young people subscribe to this and live their lives accordingly. Sadly, the Church's teaching on sex has tended to give the opposite impression, as though sex should not be fun. The negativity of this attitude was strikingly exposed by Hugh Lavery in his memorable one-liner: 'In the beginning was the word, and the word was "No"!' The fact that sex is fun is bound up with the bodily dimension of our being human persons. However, there is more to our being human persons than our bodily dimension. If we ignore the other dimensions of ourselves, particularly the relational and the social, we may discover too late that the fun we have experienced in our sexual activities is short-lived and can even dull our senses to much deeper sexual pleasures we are capable of enjoying. I could not improve on the way Moore expresses this point:

> Sex has more possibilities for pleasure and enjoyment if entered into as part of a relationship between people who mean something to each other. Those who want to treat sex purely as a matter of bodily sensations or as activities in which the identity of the partners is irrelevant or of little significance are actually missing out on a good deal of the pleasure that sex has to offer . . . In stressing the importance of personal relationship as a context for sexual activity, Christians have simply latched on to a truth about things. And they are not being strict, but trying to open themselves and others up to greater truth and greater enjoyment. (p. 62)

Here Moore is simply stressing that a sexual ethic cannot be constructed exclusively on the bodily dimension of being a human person. To attempt to do so would be to sell ourselves short as human persons.

It is sometimes argued that sexual intercourse, in itself, has no inherent meaning. It only takes on meaning through its context and that context is entirely dependent on the two people involved. It is true that, ultimately, full human meaning is dependent on the human persons involved. Hence, in any specific act of intercourse its human meaning is ultimately dependent on the two individuals concerned.

Nevertheless, sexual intercourse is not an action which is without any human significance in itself and which is totally dependent on the persons involved for its meaning.

We are our bodies. Hence, penetrative sex involves entering into a very intimate domain of a person's bodily being. It involves 'touching' a person very profoundly. To encroach upon an intimate physical domain of a person without the person's permission or invitation is a grave violation of that person's privacy. It is actually a violation of the person through a major invasion of his or her bodily being.

Because of the profundity of the intimate touching involved, sexual intercourse has the potential not only to express the love a couple have for each other but also to deepen that love or heal its wounds. On the other hand, precisely because of its profound physical intimacy, when this action is used negatively, as in rape, it is experienced by the victim as a horrendously invasive violation of her or his person. Tragically its effects can be long-term since it can seriously wound that person's capacity to experience love through intimate touching. It may not just impair the person's capacity for sustaining a loving relationship; it may actually render her or him physically insensitive to the intrinsic potential of intimate touch for mediating interpersonal love. This adds an extra dimension of horror to the evil of child sexual abuse. It can do enormous damage to the development of the child's God-given capacity to love and be loved as a sexual person.

One question which arises is whether this 'body' dimension throws any light on the issue of gay and lesbian relationships. It is argued that the bodily dimension of being a human person means that any love-making in such a relationship is bound to be incomplete and so, at best, very imperfect. This point is made by the Church of England bishops in their 1991 report *Issues in Human Sexuality*, when they write that 'there may be for some (homophiles) a mismatch between their bodies and the ways in which they wish to express their mutual self-giving' (p. 39). A similar point is made by André Guindon, in *The Sexual Creators: An Ethical Proposal for Concerned Christians* (New York, University Press of America, 1986), though he seems to have in mind more than merely biological sameness:

> The other's otherness in the male–female sexual dialogue carries within it a potential for self-discovery in one's male–female humanity which is not present in the same-sex otherness of the other . . . A lucid gay person should acknowledge the fact that the sameness of same-sex relations represents a potential deficiency in terms of other-sex challenge. (p. 169)

A few observations need to be made here about the bodily dimension of love-making in gay and lesbian relationships:

1. Although it is true that the act of penetrative sex in its heterosexual sense is not a possibility in a gay or lesbian relationship, it is also true that penetrative sex is not the only sexual expression of love. In fact, as we have already seen, for women it is often not experienced as love-making, especially when it ceases to be part of a much wider repertoire of ways of expressing love which may require much more sensitivity on the part of a man to his partner's needs and also much more mutuality. It is suggested that lesbian women and gay men have much to teach heterosexuals about the art of love-making over and above penetrative sex.

2. Guindon makes the point that same-sex relationships tend to be non-violent:

> An active non-violent style of human relationships must also be counted as a plus of the gay experience. The sameness implied in gay mutuality is, perhaps, too summarily appraised negatively. If it is true to say that sameness does not foster growth-producing conflicts, is it not equally true to state that it averts some destructive ones? . . . As Freud realised, same-sex attraction does not push gays to make war on each other but to make love to each other. (pp. 173–4)

3. Perhaps the emphasis on diversity found in the 1995 Church of England report *Something to Celebrate* has something to offer here. Diversity entails difference. Gay and lesbian sexuality is different from heterosexuality. That means that it does not offer the same relational possibilities as heterosexuality. Hence, it is limited in comparison with heterosexuality. Yet so is heterosexuality limited in comparison with homosexuality. The limitations may be different on both sides but they still remain limitations. And limitations are nothing to get worked up about. They are part of the human condition. The gift of being male or female is also a limitation. Limitations do not diminish us. They actually give a focus to our lives. Living within our limitations is not something negative. It simply means living out of our giftedness and our strengths. I believe that the discussion about homosexuality gets off on the wrong footing when homosexuals try to argue that homosexuality is good in all the same ways that heterosexuality is good. It would be better if homosexuals and heterosexuals were prepared to accept that, in this aspect of their sexuality, they are simply different from each other. That is another way of recognizing their respective

limitations. To be different is not to be second-class or inferior. To be different is not to be objectively disordered. It is simply to be different. Difference only becomes a disorder when it involves a propensity to behave in a way which contradicts respect for the dignity of the human person. That would be the case in paedophilia, for instance.

4. One of the myths about gays is that they have a propensity towards paedophilia. This myth fuels still further the fires of homo-phobia and leads to discriminatory practice against gays. In his book *Slayer of the Soul: Child Sexual Abuse and the Catholic Church* (Connecticut, Twenty-Third Publications, 1991), Stephen J. Rossetti mentions a vocation director justifying non-acceptance of gay men as candidates for his religious congregation because of 'all this paedophilia stuff that is going on'. He even quotes the renowned religious sociologist, Andrew Greeley, as saying: 'Most homosexuals are not paedophiles and some paedophiles are not homosexual. Nonetheless, the two phenomena shade into one another' (p. 11). Rossetti refutes such allegations by quoting a variety of scientific studies. One concluded that 'homosexuality and homosexual paedophilia may be mutually exclusive and that the adult heterosexual male constitutes a greater risk to the underage child than does the adult homosexual male'. This was recognized in *An Introduction to the Pastoral Care of Homosexual People*, produced in 1979 by the Catholic Social Welfare Commission of the Bishops' Conference of England and Wales: 'In fact, it would seem that proportionately to their numbers in the population, the hetero-sexuals are more prone to child molestation than homosexuals' (p. 5, sub-heading b). The Catholic bishops of Washington State said something similar in their 1983 policy document *The Prejudice against Homosexuals and the Ministry of the Church*: 'A number of Catholics are concerned about the role of homosexuals in professions which have the care of children. There are those who think gays and lesbians inevitably impart a homosexual value system to children or that they will molest children. This is a prejudice and must be unmasked as such. There is no evidence that exposure to homosexuals, of itself, harms a child' (full text in Jeannine Gramick and Robert Nugent, *Voices of Hope: A Collection of Positive Catholic Writings on Gay and Lesbian Issues*, New York, Center for Homophobia Education, 1995, pp. 89–97, at p. 97). Another study quoted by Rossetti notes that the phenomenon of paedophilia is linked not to sexual orientation but to having problems in 'establishing satisfactory adult relationships'. A further study reports that many child sexual abusers would identify themselves as heterosexual, even if they have been involved with children of the

same sex, and notes that this appears to be especially true of priests and the religious (p. 12).

5. THE GIFTEDNESS OF HUMAN LIFE

Like 'pro choice', the phrase 'pro life' has been hi-jacked by one side in the abortion debate. In that context, 'life' is meant to denote unborn life, life in the womb. Defence of unborn life is made a moral absolute. From the moment of conception life is considered to be sacrosanct. Leaving aside some of the assumptions of this position which are not beyond challenge and debate, to limit the meaning of life in this way does not do justice to the wider concern for life which lies at the heart of Christian ethics. The late Cardinal Joseph Bernardin pointed this out repeatedly in his many challenging addresses on the theme of 'the consistent life-ethic'. A collection of these addresses, along with some of the discussion they provoked, is found in his book *Consistent Ethic of Life* (Kansas City, Sheed & Ward, 1988).

My use of the phrase 'pro life' as describing an essential dimension of Christian sexual ethics is more in line with Bernardin's interpretation. Perhaps it is even more inclusive than his use of the phrase. Ultimately, being 'pro life' is about being committed to life as something much bigger than ourselves. It is recognizing that, as human persons, we are essentially social beings. Consequently, when it comes to the sphere of sexual ethics, the 'pro life' dimension of our being sexual beings should not be reduced to the procreational potentiality of human sexuality, even though that is an important aspect of it. It is certainly true that children are a social concern – the future of society ultimately depends on them. Yet the social dimension of our being sexual persons goes far beyond the birth and upbringing of children. We are interdependent, relational beings and just how far-reaching is our social interdependence is something which the science of sociology is bringing home to us, as we have already seen in Chapter Two. Just as we are not persons living in our bodies, so we are not persons living *in* society; we are human persons *through* living in society. The social dimension is part of our being human. Understanding 'pro life' in this broader sense, it must be said that we are being inhuman if we refuse to be 'pro life'.

Our sexuality is part of the 'pro life' thrust of our being. It draws us into life since it pushes us out of our isolation and attracts us to other people. The relational dimension of our sexuality is already 'pro life', even before we consider its procreational dimension. As mentioned in Chapter Five, the Churches have taken this on board and now recognize that marriage is primarily a covenant relationship of love rather than simply an institution to serve the procreation of children. Hence, children are referred to as the 'fruit' rather than the *raison d'être* of their parents' love.

Nevertheless, it is very noticeable that the Churches, while realigning the relationship between love and procreation, still insist that they are inseparably connected, despite disagreements as to how this insepar-able connection is to be honoured. For instance, in the previous chapter we saw how the Roman Catholic Church and the Church of England, though disagreeing about how the inseparable connection between the relational and the procreational dimensions should be present in the sexual activity of a married couple, both agree that the connection between these dimensions is inseparable. The Roman Catholic position maintains that it must be respected in every sexual act to the extent that nothing must be done to nullify the procreational potential of the act. The Church of England position, on the other hand, holds that it is sufficient for the procreational dimension to be embodied in the relationship itself. When that is the case, individual acts, even if physically contraceptive, still belong to the procreative project of the marriage itself.

Perhaps the deeper truth which the Churches are absolutely committed to here is the inseparable connection between love and life. Love is a powerful life-giving force. If we fail to love, we dry up as human persons. Our life begins to wither. Because of the insepar-ablility of love and life, this same truth can be expressed the other way round. If we do not open ourselves to life, our capacity to love will wither. If we are not open to other people, we are not open to life.

In using 'pro life' in this broader sense I am not suggesting that the procreational dimension of 'pro life' is something which is the concern only of those who decide to have children. It is a concern which involves all of us, married or celibate, heterosexual or homosexual. Specifically as sexual persons we are all called to be loving women and men. Because of the inseparable connection between sexual love and procreation, our lives as loving persons must embody real respect for this procreative dimension. Although it seems true that, the higher up the evolutionary ladder a species is, the more sexuality seems to take on a relational capacity as well as being procreational, nevertheless, the procreational dimension remains fundamental to our sexuality.

Since our sexuality is part of the social dimension of our being human persons, we all share in a joint responsibility for ensuring the continued survival of our species by parenting the children of the next generation. This joint responsibility is part of our self-identity as human persons. In a sense, each of us, as current members of the human family, must be committed to the survival of our species. As human persons, we have no right to say that future generations are not our concern. We would actually be denying our self-identity as human persons if we disowned concern for procreation as an essential dimension of who we are.

I believe that this social commitment to child-bearing and parent-hood can be present in the lives of people who will never be parents in much the same way as the Church of England believes the procreative dimension of marriage can be present in sexual acts which are biologically contraceptive. In other words, precisely because we are social persons, the lives of those of us who will never be parents can still be seen as having meaning in terms of a commitment to the survival of our human species. Let me explain what I mean by that.

As individual members of the human species, each of us needs to own the procreative dimension of human sexuality, on which the survival of our species depends. To disown it would be to opt out of being human, since it would be to deny an essential part of our self-identity as social persons. However, to accept procreation as a basic human value does not mean that we ourselves necessarily have to be directly involved in the procreative process. We can own the procreative dimension of our human sexuality without feeling obliged ourselves to bring children into the world. For instance, an acceptance of the procreative dimension of human sexuality needs to be part of the fundamental mind-set of people like myself who have embraced a celibate life and so will never procreate offspring. The same is true of most lifelong single people and also of married couples who, whether by accident or choice, do not have children.

What about people, if such there be, who totally reject the idea that we have any communal social obligation to continue our human species or who very deliberately refuse to accept it as any concern of theirs? Any individual or couple adopting that approach to life would seem to be opting out of an important part of what it means to be truly human. They would be disowning an essential element in the social dimension of being a human person. In a sense, at the wider social level they would be denying the inseparable link between procreation and human sexuality. They would be saying that for them human sexuality has no meaning apart from the relational or recreational. That would be tantamount to saying that procreation is purely an optional extra and has nothing to do with what it means to be human.

Lisa Cahill would detect a flavour of this approach in the too-blinkered approach to freedom found among some liberal thinkers. Her fear is that, in their desire to free the human spirit from all constraints, they are prepared to break away from what is, in fact, an absolutely essential dimension of our being human persons, namely, our corporeality. She discusses this in her essay 'On the connection of sex to reproduction', in Earl Shelp (ed.), *Sexuality and Medicine: vol. II, Ethical Viewpoints in Transition* (Dordrecht, Kluwer Academic Publishers, 1987), pp. 39–50. For her there is no getting away from the fact that our reproductive capacity is part of our bodiliness and has profound implications for who we are as relational and social beings. She fully recognizes that personhood is more distinctively human than our human reproductive biological faculties. Hence, it is entirely right that human 'freedom and rationality control and direct biology and the physical conditions of life in community' (p. 43). However, liberalism goes much further than that: 'In the liberal view, individuals are seen as free agents who are not intrinsically interdependent and related through innate social and moral bonds, but who enter into "consenting adult" relationships wherein they agree to duties of noninterference or of reciprocal support in the pursuit of their own ends'. Our reproductive biology becomes, therefore, not something we 'control and direct' but something to be 'liberated from'. For Cahill this is a serious failure to appreciate fully our corporeality which, after all, is 'a precondition of the sexual relationship as interpersonal, and an essential dimension of sexual experience and sexual acts themselves' (p. 44). For her, liberalism is essentially reductionist in its approach to the human person and this leads it to be equally reductionist with regard to the human community:

> The sexual capacity of the human body is just as obviously conducive to reproduction as it is to reciprocal sexual pleasure. The meaning of human sexual function as embodied is not exhausted by affective and emotional and physical satisfaction, though those are essential constituents of its meaning, and perhaps even the most important ones. The fullness of the human sexual reality is neglected if we simply overlook in normative analysis the fact that the creation of offspring is one 'natural' purpose of sex as a physical phenomenon, and that the consolidation of a relationship (the conjugal and parental one), and of a social group conducive to the nurturance and education of offspring (the family) are among the purposes for which the affective and interpersonal dimensions of sexuality are apt. The

intergenerational family (which can and does assume many forms in many cultures) is a physical and interpersonal structure of connection between the sexuality of the individual and the community. As others have noted, it is communal interdependence, in both its physical or material and interpersonal aspects, which is critically neglected in 'liberal' accounts of human nature. (pp. 44–5)

What Cahill is objecting to is liberalism's assumption that the cause of human freedom is to be advanced through humankind's being liberated from our generative biological processes. Far from being a liberation, she sees that as discarding an important dimension of our being human. However, this does not imply that the essential connection between sex and reproduction provides a clear-cut ethical imperative for the relationships and acts of every individual couple: 'Since intimacy is a more distinctively human meaning of sex than procreation, the latter is a secondary good in relation to the former and may for sufficient reason be eliminated from a particular sex act, or even from the relationship as a whole' (p. 48). Cahill does not accept the Pope's position on contraception. She has no problem with the responsible use of contraception. However, she totally rejects any position which holds that the reproductive significance of human sexuality is simply an optional extra for people who might be interested in that kind of thing. For Cahill, the connection between sex and reproduction is part of our human make-up. We throw it overboard at our peril.

What are the implications of the connection between sex and reproduction for same-sex relationships? One major objection raised against same-sex activity is that it is not open to procreation. At a purely biological level that cannot be denied. Nor can it be claimed that the procreational significance of same-sex activity is supplied by the overall relationship itself, since that too is not procreative in the strict sense of the word. However, as individuals and as couples, gay men and lesbian women can still be 100 per cent committed to the human family's procreative enterprise. By using their own creative gifts, often highly developed, they can contribute very substantially to the enrichment and survival of the human species. As mentioned above, the procreative enterprise, in its holistic sense, is about far more than providing for the survival of the species by giving birth to children. It is also about the qualitative survival of the species. Therefore, it is also involves passing on to future generations the benefits of a rich culture.

It is sometimes objected that for society to adopt a positive attitude towards gay and lesbian relationships would pose a threat to marriage. This is a strange objection. It gives the impression that the procreative enterprise is experienced by the human family as an enormous burden and that everyone is simply longing to be freed from this burden, given half an excuse. I do not believe that is true. I suspect that kind of fear is based on another version of dualist thinking. It makes the human sexual drive too cerebral and ignores our glorious oneness with the animal kingdom. Our sexual drive is part of our survival instinct as a species. That is not lost when it is raised to the higher plane of communicating interpersonal love. Perhaps the real threat to truly human marriage and the survival of our species does not come from gays or lesbians but from those heterosexual couples mentioned above whose understanding of marriage is so impoverished that they believe it has no other meaning or purpose than their own personal happiness. That turns marriage into an *égoïsme à deux*. Such an attitude is both anti-social and anti-life. It certainly has no place in a Christian sexual ethics.

We are frequently reminded that marriage is meant to be for life. That brings up another meaning of 'for life' of great importance in sexual ethics. The phrase 'for life' resonates with the notion of lifelong faithfulness. Earlier in this chapter we have seen how a commitment to a lifelong relationship, far from being an abdication of freedom, is actually an exercise of freedom at its highest level. It involves an act of faith in what we are capable of as persons endowed with free will.

I share the belief, which we heard expressed by the Churches in the previous chapter, that 'for life' is an essential dimension of the relationship-building process that a committed couple have pledged themselves to. Without this 'for life' dimension the process is doomed to failure. Lest this claim be misunderstood, I would like to stress that, in making it, I am not claiming that 'for life' commitments cannot fail. Tragically, they can and they do. Nor am I suggesting that a 'for life' commitment is just another word for marriage. There are some very inspirational 'for life' relationships among cohabiting couples. Likewise, there are marriages in which the couples involved have made no real commitment to build a 'for life' commitment between them. Moreover, I am not implying that building a 'for life' relationship is simply a matter of determination and will-power. I do not believe that for a moment. Jack Dominian has shown very clearly that building a 'for life' relationship will involve a couple in a mutual growth process across a number of different dimensions of life. For a variety of reasons, some developmental, some external, and many of them quite outside their control, a couple may not be able to engage properly with this process or bring it to fruition. Nor do I believe that 'for life' relationships cannot be prepared for by more transitory relationships. Youth has always been a kind of transition time in life when experience in relating to others is gained through the joys and pains of exploring passing friendships. In reality, some so-called 'for life' marriages would fit better into this category of exploratory, transitory relationships.

For love to take root and grow, trust is needed. For trust to develop, intimacy needs to grow between a couple. This in turn involves increasing vulnerability as they open themselves out to each other and accept each other through the process of mutual disclosure. What they are sharing in such loving intimacy is their very selves. That is impossible without mutual trust. Not every intimate relationship involves the sharing of sexual intimacy between the couple. Where it does, however, mutual trust is essential if such sexual sharing is to be a sharing of persons.

6. THE UNIQUENESS OF THE HUMAN PERSON AND RESPECT FOR PERSONAL CONSCIENCE

Each of us is not just an individual instance of the genus, human person. We are all unique. And the paradox is that this uniqueness is an essential dimension of being human that we all share in common. This unique dimension of the human person has been coming very much to the fore in recent years. It is one of the key emphases in postmodernism. (At the time of writing this chapter it has even been raised as a factor in the debate over human cloning.) At a very profound level of our person we are all different from each other. If we are to respond to the human dignity of our fellow human beings, we need to respect the 'otherness' of each person. We must not confine the 'other' by completely reducing him or her to our own predetermined categories. There is always a radical heart to each person which lies beyond definition.

Nevertheless, our uniqueness as human persons is only one dimension of our being human. Nor can it exist in isolation from the other dimensions. It permeates them all. For instance, there is something unique about the way we embrace our freedom as well as about our bodies, our personal and social relationships, our personal histories and especially our relationship with God. Our uniqueness is not some kind of residue left behind when we have filtered out everything we share in common with other persons. Our uniqueness as human persons can only grow and develop through the way each of us embraces and lives out positively these other dimensions of our humanness. And we will each do that in our own unique way.

1. To your own self be true

Our uniqueness is part of our giftedness. I receive myself as gift, as responsibility, as vocation. I am called to be myself, not someone else. It is this over-arching transcendental context of my existing as pure gift which gives the lie to any interpretation which would claim that my uniqueness constitutes utter self-sufficiency and absolute autonomy. Ultimately I am not my own. I am untrue to my uniqueness when I try to cut myself adrift from my createdness and go into a kind of free-fall. Then my uniqueness loses the comforting richness of being a gift and I am left with the terrifying aloneness of isolation and alienation.

Personal uniqueness is also tied in with our freedom and responsibility. Not only do I have to accept personal responsibility for my moral decisions. I also have to ensure that my moral decisions really are *my own* decisions. Consequently, I cannot shift on to another person – or institution – either the responsibility for the decisions I have made or *the actual making* of those decisions. When I decide that such and such an action is what I must do, it must be I myself who am making that decision. That is not to deny that there may be many occasions when I decide to heed the advice of others or when I obey the legitimate directives of someone who has authority over me and whose authority I respect. In such cases I am still the one who is making this decision about myself, provided I am not abdicating personal responsibility by acting out of unthinking blind obedience or slavishly following teaching I do not believe in.

Acknowledging our uniqueness does not mean that each of us is a law unto ourselves. General norms play an essential role in our lives. Such norms are based on what we share in common as human persons. However, they are not the whole picture. Our moral sensitivity and our conscience comprise much more than a mere down-loading of universal moral principles into our mind's ethical data system. They will have been formed and coloured by our own unique personal experience. This ongoing, experience-based formation process will also have been affected by the various people who have played an important part in our lives and particularly in our moral education. The result of the combined influence of such people and many other factors, including our family and cultural background, will be the moral sensitivity and conscience which are unique to each of us.

It is important to note that there is a link between uniqueness and difference and how they feature in a person-centred sexual ethics. Obviously, they do not mean the same thing. John is a unique person but that is not because he is a man and not a woman, or because he is gay and not heterosexual. His maleness and his gayness make him different from many other people but they do not make him unique. In a sense, uniqueness could be described as difference writ large. Our uniqueness makes us different, not just from many other human persons, but from every other human person.

At the heart of morality lies respect for 'the other'. The other is different from us. That difference lies most fundamentally in his or her uniqueness, but it also lies in those more general characteristics in which his or her uniqueness is incarnate and which we do not all share. Fundamentally, John is different from Mary because he is John, and not Mary. However, part of his difference is that he is a man and Mary is a woman. Therefore, in respecting a person's uniqueness, we are also called to respect his or her difference from us.

Of course, this is not denying the fundamental principles of morality as they are derived from our shared belief in the dignity of the human person and from those basic dimensions of being a human person which we all share in common. John might be unique in the particular way he sexually abuses children. That does not mean that my respect for his uniqueness as a human person demands that I have to approve of his child sexual abuse. Sexual abuse of any kind, but especially when children are the victims, is a violation of the basic humanity which John and I and every other human person share in common. What we are called to recognize and respect is the unique package of giftedness and woundedness that each of us is and also the unique way in which an individual is able to positively integrate this package of light and shade in the various dimensions of being a human person. Consequently, in no way are we called to respect the unique way in which an individual might deliberately give up working at any such integration and instead opt out of behaving as a human person through a serious violation of the common humanity he or she shares with all other people.

In Chapter Four (pp. 86–7) I stressed that my whole approach to homosexuality followed in this book is based on the assumption that it is true, as the 1982 Methodist Working Party report claims, that '(homosexual persons) are as capable as other people . . . of deeply loving and committed relationships with each other' and that there is no scientific evidence to support the many myths which present homosexual persons as a danger either to themselves or other persons or to the moral health of a nation. Granted that is the case, then a person's homosexual orientation can be embraced as part of his or her giftedness and celebrated accordingly. For the Christian, therefore, it is part of the giftedness which a person should be drawn to thank God for. This is not to deny, as has also been mentioned in Chapter Four, that, in practice, the attitude of Church and society to homosexuality might mean that this gift comes to an individual in a damaged condition and may even be experienced as a form of woundedness. The healing 'good news' of the Christian Gospel is not that this gift of homosexual orientation can be reversed but that it can be accepted by this person as part of his or her unique package of giftedness. Clearly the same cannot be said of any sexual predisposition which inclines a person to act harmfully towards others or oneself. While that predisposition needs to be 'owned' as part of the 'wounded' side of one's unique package as a person, the importance of 'owning' it lies in the fact that this opens out the possibility of getting appropriate help either towards healing or, at least, to achieving a lifestyle which makes one less of a danger to others and oneself.

2. Respect for conscience: personal goodness is not synonymous with ethical rightness

In his book *Moral Demands and Personal Obligations* (Washington, Georgetown University Press, 1993), the German moral theologian Josef Fuchs states: 'The distinction is made today between the ethical goodness of the person – morality in the truest sense of the word – and the *ethical rightness* of action or behaviour.' (p. 157; emphasis original). For Fuchs 'the ethical goodness of the person' is 'morality in the truest sense of the word' because it is dealing with the inner integrity of a person. That is why it goes to the heart of a person-centred approach to moral theology.

In the area of practical decision-making what is meant by 'ethical goodness' is that a person tries to honour his or her personal integrity in the reality of everyday life to the best of their ability. They do this if they have *with openness and integrity* tried their best to discern what course of action in their particular circumstances and taking account of their personal moral capacity is most in keeping with the criterion of the dignity of the human person, integrally and adequately considered – *a criterion to which they are fully committed.* They realize that their judgement is fallible and so it is possible that they are mistaken. Nevertheless, as long as they have made a serious conscientious judgement according to their best lights, they have clearly demonstrated their commitment to personal integrity.

Within the Roman Catholic Church, for instance, this means that no official teaching on sexual ethics can oblige a Catholic to act against their conscience or to accept as true any ethical ruling of the Church which they conscientiously believe not to be true. It also means that a person is abdicating their moral responsibility as a human person if they decline to follow their own convinced conscience purely because a Church directive on sexual ethics forbids them to do what they know they really should do.

This is not saying anything which is contrary to what Roman Catholic moral theology has always taught. It is merely drawing out an important truth regarding conformity to the Church's moral teaching which is implicit in two items of traditional teaching. This truth is that being in conformity with official Church teaching has never been accepted as an adequate criterion either (1) for assessing an individual's 'personal goodness' in decision-making or (2) for assessing the ethical rightness of an action. Conclusion (1) above follows from the accepted teaching that a person must always be faithful to his or her conscience, even when it is inculpably erroneous. Although this teaching was usually expressed by saying that a person following such a conscience was not blameworthy, implicit in the teaching was the acknowledgement that such a person was, in fact, praiseworthy in being faithful to their personal integrity. This is simply another way of saying that personal goodness is found in being faithful to one's conscience, even when it is inculpably in error. Conclusion (2) flows from the traditional teaching that the respect due to authoritative non-infallible moral teaching in the Church does not totally rule out the possibility of responsible disagreement. I have explored this further in my book *New Directions in Moral Theology* (cf. Epilogue, 'Dialogue, diversity and truth: the vocation of the moral theologian in the Roman Catholic Church today', pp. 138–59) and also in my article 'Conformity and dissent in the Church', in *The Way*, 1988, pp. 87–101. Hence, the possibility of responsible disagreement means that whether a person's decision is in conformity with official Church teaching is not an adequate criterion for assessing 'personal moral goodness' in decision-making. It is not even an adequate criterion for assessing the 'ethical rightness' of the action being done. Although traditional moral theology held that there should be a 'presumption' in favour of the truth of that teaching, nevertheless, as Richard McCormick points out, that presumption is 'weakened' if those proposing the teaching have short-circuited the process and have not 'appropriately tapped the available sources of human understanding' ('The search for truth in the Catholic context', in *America*, 8 November 1986, p. 278).

Hence, if a couple are convinced that the Church's official teaching on contraception is erroneous, they are not obliged to accept this teaching as true. In fact, they would be wrong to do so while they remain in their present state of mind. If they go on to decide that the good of their own marriage dictates they should use contraception themselves, they should regard their decision as well taken and so they can rest assured that they remain pleasing to God. The same would hold even for a couple who are in substantial agreement with the Church's teaching on contraception. If they have reached a conscientious decision that, all things considered (including the Church's teaching), the good of their marriage and their family requires them to use some form of contraception, once again they should regard their decision as well taken and they too can feel at peace with God. Something similar would hold true across the board in the whole field of sexual ethics. So, for instance, it would also apply to similar conscientious decision-making on the part of of gay men and lesbian women expressing their love sexually in a committed, faithful relationship or cohabiting heterosexual couples or people entering a second marriage after divorce.

In none of these cases is it a matter of people just doing whatever they like in any trivial sense. As mentioned above, I am assuming that we are dealing with people who do not have a purely self-centred agenda. They are committed to trying to be faithful to the basic moral criterion of the dignity of the human person, integrally and adequately considered. They are also trying to behave responsibly both in the ongoing task of conscience-formation and in how they go about their conscientious decision-making. That being the case, in all these instances people are obliged to follow their conscientious judgement as to what is the right thing to do; and this remains true, even when their conscientious judgement seems to be at odds with Church teaching.

To express this in theological language, a person following their conscience in this way can be absolutely certain that, in so doing, they are not deviating from their commitment to be faithful to God's will. Put very simply, they are doing the best they can and God does not ask for more. In following their conscience in this way, they are being 'ethically good' as persons, even though it is possible that what they are doing might not be 'ethically right'.

3. The uniqueness of each person's story of moral growth

Our striving to live a good moral life will be profoundly influenced by where we are at as persons at this moment. Clearly, therefore, it will be affected by our level of sexual, psychological and spiritual development. For most of us such personal development does not follow an orderly progression through precisely defined stages over a period of time. Rather it embraces all the ups and downs of our unique and often very unpredictable personal stories. The story of some people's lives can be very turbulent indeed. It might include deeply wounding experiences such as being abused as a child, or the separation of one's parents, or the breakdown of one's marriage, or subjection to physical violence or even rape, or drug or alcohol dependence, or sudden and tragic bereavement. Such experiences will have a major impact on an individual person's unique life-story and on his or her capacity to cope with the demands of interpersonal or social relationships. Understandably, such experiences will often have a negative impact on an individual's personal development, though, paradoxically, with loving and patient support they can sometimes be turned into positive growth points in a person's life. Hopefully, the story of most people's lives is principally made up of experiences which help to develop their capacity to cope with life. These growth factors have a bearing on personal goodness. Personal goodness is about being true to ourselves *at our present stage of growth in moral development.*

A person-centred sexual ethics accepts that growth is a sign of life and is part of the God-given reality we have to grapple with. Growth in moral maturity and understanding is a sign of life not just in individual persons but also in institutions, including the Churches. In Chapter Five we saw how the Churches have, in fact, grown in wisdom and understanding with regard to the sexual dimension of being a human person made in the image of God. And this process is still going on.

In his 1981 Apostolic Exhortation on 'The Role of the Christian Family in the Modern World' (*Familiaris Consortio*), n. 34, John Paul II writes: 'What is known as "the law of gradualness" or step-by-step advance cannot be identified with "gradualness of the law", as if there were different degrees or forms of precept in God's law for different individuals and situations.' The Pontifical Council for the Family quote this to support their own similar statement: 'The pastoral "law of gradualness", not to be confused with the "gradualness of the law" which would tend to diminish the demands it places on us, consists of requiring a decisive break with sin together with a progressive path towards total union with the will of God and with his loving demands' ('Vademecum for confessors on some themes of conjugal morality', in *Briefing*, 20 March 1997, n. 9, p. 37). What they mean by the 'gradualness of the law' is not clear. Certainly, a person-centred morality believes in a law of 'growth' which is not about 'diminishing' God's demands on us but about discerning the 'progressive path' we are called to follow as unique human persons. Doing the best we can today may be a necessary stage in our becoming empowered to do even better tomorrow.

In no way would a person-centred sexual ethics want to deny that *what we do* matters in the eyes of God. Virtually all our actions affect other persons and they, like us, are precious to God. Yet what matters at least equally to God is *our own personal goodness (or lack of it)* which is mediated through our other-affecting behaviour. As Fuchs says in the passage quoted earlier, that is 'morality in the truest sense of the word'. Our *personal goodness* and *what we do* are related to each other. Yet there is a certain ambiguity in the equation between them. At times, what we do is a very revealing expression of who we are as a person; at other times, what we do conceals the 'real me'; and at other times what we do shapes who we are becoming as a person. The mystery and ambiguity of human becoming is overlooked if we reduce the meaning of 'objective morality' simply to *what a person does* and leave out of the equation *where the person is at who is doing the action*. That is not being truly 'objective' since it only presents a partial picture of what is going on. Russell B. Connors calls such a partial presentation morally 'thin' because it fails to ask some key 'reality revealing questions' about what is going on. Borrowing terminology from Clifford Geertz and Gilbert Ryle, he argues that only a 'thick' presentation which takes account of both the commonality and particularity of moral experience can give a true picture of our moral living (cf. Russell B. Connors, 'Thick and thin: an angle on Catholic moral teaching', in *Louvain Studies*,

1996, pp. 336–55). In my article 'Moral theology in the parish', in *Priests and People*, 1994, pp. 367–72, I use different language to make the same point:

> It might help to go back to the parable of the wheat and the darnel. Normative ethics helps us to recognise both wheat and darnel. However, the owner of the field is doing something other than recognising their joint presence in his field . . . He has faith in the healthy growth of his wheat, despite all the darnel mixed in with it. His principal concern is to protect his wheat from the misguided zeal of those intent on destroying the darnel without any regard for the harm this might do to the wheat. Normative ethics is moral theology in its role of distinguishing right from wrong . . . Pastorally, (it can) be like the beautiful picture found on the outside of a seed packet. It can motivate us to plant the seed in the first place. But part of the pastoral role of moral theology is to help the seed to grow, despite soil deficiency, adverse weather, surrounding weeds and lots of other threatening dangers. . . . Moral theology is not meant to condemn the plant emerging from the seed simply because it does not live up to the promise of the idealised picture on the packet. Rather it appreciates the growth that occurs. Sometimes what might look like a puny and undeveloped plant might, in fact, be a miracle of growth, given the adverse conditions under which it has had to struggle. (pp. 370–1)

7

SEXUALITY AND SIN

SEX IS NOT SINFUL: IT IS A GIFT OF GOD

For most of the Church's history Christian sexual ethics tended to give the impression that human sexuality was a dimension of our personal life inextricably bound up with sin. Today the picture is changing. Christians are more and more acknowledging that sexuality is something to be celebrated. It is an important dimension of our gifted-ness by God. We see human sexuality in particular as having special significance and dignity since it is an essential dimension of ourselves as relational persons, made in the image of a relational God. Our sexu-ality fuels our drive for connectedness with others. Openness to life is not limited to the procreational potential of our sexuality. It is our sexual energy which impels us to go beyond a self-centred existence and involve ourselves with others, interpersonally and socially, in the ongoing creation and celebration of life. Audre Lorde calls this the 'power of the erotic'. Her oft-quoted essay 'Uses of the erotic: the erotic as power' (in *Sister Outsider: Essays and Speeches*, Trumansburg, NY, Crossing Press, 1984, pp. 52–9) reads like a hymn of thanks and praise for the wonderful and powerful gift of our sexuality.

Many people say that we are living in an age plagued by eroticism. The media and advertising agencies are inundating us with erotic images. Lorde would claim that this is confusing the erotic with the pornographic which, in her view, is a 'direct denial of the power of the erotic, for it represents the suppression of true feeling' and, in fact, 'emphasizes sensation without feeling' (p. 54). She suggests that the problem with our age is that the influence of manipulative power has suppressed the erotic in our lives with the result that our lives are lived mostly at the level of the trivial and without any real creative energy.

Lorde believes that women are once more getting in touch with the creative power of the erotic. Being in touch with that power can energize all of us, men as well as women, to 'pursue genuine change within our world' (p. 59).

To see our sexuality as something to be celebrated does not mean that it is a dimension of our lives that is immune from sin. No area of human life carries such immunity. Sin is to be found in the sexual dimension of our lives just as much as it is in all the other dimensions. However, it is not sex that makes a person sinful. It is the person that can make sex sinful. Hence, sin must not be identified with the sexual dimension itself. Sex is not sinful. It is a good gift of God. What is sinful is the way human persons can behave destructively towards themselves and others in the sexual domain. The criterion for what is sinful in the sexual field is exactly the same as for any other area of our lives. What is sinful is what violates the good of the human person, integrally and adequately considered.

PATRIARCHY AS SEXUAL SIN – AND THE SEXUAL SIN OF COLLUSION IN PATRIARCHY

Our sexuality touches a very profound level of our being human persons. The sexual violation of a person does not just affect his or her body. It affects them precisely as persons. It is the person who is raped, or abused, or dehumanized by being turned into a commercial object for some consumer's use. Whenever a person is 'de-personalized' by being used merely as the object of another's sexual gratification or displaced aggression, we are faced with a grave instance of sin in the sexual field. A person-centred Christian sexual ethics will see this as a terrible abuse of sexuality rather than as due to any innate sinfulness in sexuality itself.

In Chapter Six we saw that a Christian sexual ethics which is truly person-centred needs to be specifically pro-women in this time in which we are living. For such a person-centred sexual ethic patriarchy must surely be recognized as a structural sin of the highest gravity in the area of sexuality. To the extent that we as individuals or institutions willingly collude in patriarchal structures, we have to bear some share of responsibility for the continued existence of this structural sexual sin. That being so, it follows that the Churches, to the extent that they fail to dissociate themselves from such collusion and combat the sexual injustice of patriarchy, stand guilty of sexual sin.

The impact of such a conclusion is sometimes softened by the assertion that, though the Church might be involved in the structural sin of patriarchy, this does not mean that individual church-people are personally responsible for this sinful state of affairs. That assertion needs to be questioned. 'Sin' is a theological word. It reminds us that God is affected by what is happening. It is a very reductionist approach to sin to suggest that God is not affected by structural sin since no personal guilt is involved and so God is not actually offended by anyone.

In fact, structural sin is far from being unimportant in the eyes of God. If God really loves people and wants them to love and respect each other, it matters enormously to God how we treat each other and how we manage the world that we share as our communal home. God is not an impartial judge passing guilty or not-guilty verdicts on people. God is a committed and deeply involved lover to whom the dignity and happiness of each of us is of crucial importance. God's gracious love for us has made God very vulnerable since, like any lover, God suffers in and through the sufferings of the beloved. To look on structural sin as not really sin and, therefore, unimportant can breed an attitude of irresponsibility towards life. It seems to reduce our present life to a kind of waiting-room for eternity, a supporting feature before the main film. By putting the emphasis on my personal immunity from guilt, it seems to suggest that, as long as my conscience is clear, I do not need to worry about how the lives of other people are affected.

Futhermore, the assertion that there is nothing 'personal' about structural sin needs to challenged. It is simply not true. If we believe that sin is not caused by God or by any demonic agency, we have to recognize that human agency lies at the root of all sin. Sometimes the human agent is an individual person; sometimes it might be a group of persons or even a whole community; and sometimes it might be some kind of human structure or institution. However, in this last case such human structures are never completely free-standing. They are human artefacts and they are sustained by the collaboration of the mass of individual persons involved. When such structures or institutions are called 'sinful', human agency is still involved. It is located in the mass of human persons colluding in them. John Paul II makes this point very forcefully in his encyclical *Sollicitudo Rei Socialis* (1987): ' . . . it is not out of place to speak of "structures of sin" which . . . are rooted in personal sin, and thus always linked to the concrete acts of individuals who introduce these structures, consolidate them and make them difficult to remove. And thus they grow stronger, spread, and become the source of other sins, and so influence people's behaviour' (n. 36).

It is surely noteworthy that, as portrayed in the Gospels, the greatest obstacle Jesus encountered was the blindness of powerful people with regard to the structural sin they were upholding and which was literally imprisoning the 'poor' and the 'sinners' through a distorted interpretation of their relationship with God. Jesus was concerned to free the poor from this imprisonment – but he also struggled, with little success, to break through the blindness of their religious leaders.

Conversion in the case of structural sin is not just about breaking the bonds of institutionalized injustice, even though that is an integral element of the proclamation of the Gospel (cf. 1971 Rome Synod, *Justice in the World*, p. 6). It is also about opening the eyes of those colluding in these sinful structures. Presumably this conversion process involves a dawning recognition on the part of these collaborators that they have been colluding in a horrendous sin. Such a recognition will arouse feelings of utter horror in them. Their reaction flowing from their conversion will not be: 'So what! I was not aware of the sin I was colluding in, so I'm not guilty.' Rather it will be: 'How awful! To think that I have played a part in upholding such a dehumanizing situation.' That realization is why they feel a need for forgiveness – and also why they will be overjoyed to find that this forgiveness is given freely by God. Consequently, there is a very real sense in which structural sin is personal sin.

The victims of structural sin are often the ones branded as sinners. In fact, this is merely compounding the injustice. In many cases they are people whose options have been so reduced by structural injustice that they are struggling to live as humanly as possible within such personally destructive situations. Moreover, the irony is that they, too, often feel a need for what they mistakenly call 'forgiveness'. However, for them this so-called 'forgiveness' has a different feel about it and the route to it is very different. It is found in the realization that they have done nothing that needs forgiveness. They are loved uncondi-tionally by God just as they are. Nevertheless, if there is nothing in them that needs forgiveness, tragically there may well be much in them that needs healing. Paradoxically, their woundedness makes them all the more precious to God, as Jesus made abundantly clear. The route to their healing can be a long and hard one, as anyone knows who has ever accompanied such a person along the way. Because our sexuality involves our potentiality for being connected in love with others, the experience of being abused sexually can seriously sever that connection and displace its love potential with a paralysing fear. The hurt of sexual violation can so wound sexuality's potentiality for connectedness that such a person retreats into isolation until the wound gradually begins to heal. Such a wound rarely heals of its own accord. It needs the kind of love in another which, like the love of Jesus, is prepared to be crucified along the way before resurrection occurs.

'DOING THE BEST ONE CAN' IN SEXUAL ETHICS

What was said in the sixth section of the previous chapter with regard to 'doing the best one can' has important implications for what is meant by sin. It is particularly important in the area of sexual sin. One of David Lodge's first novels was entitled *How Far Can You Go?* It was a humorous critique of the approach to sexual morality engendered among many Catholics in the 1950s by the moral theology of their day. It was as though the demarcation lines between what was right or wrong in sexual behaviour had to be spelt out with the utmost precision since there were no half measures in the area of sexuality. According to the accepted wisdom nothing was 'light matter'. Every sexual sin qualified as grave, given the required knowledge and consent. Moreover, what was looked on as sinful (and gravely so) was any enjoyment of sexual pleasure outside of marriage. From such a starting point it was virtually impossible to arrive at any kind of interim growth sexual ethics which could help or encourage an adolescent passing through the developmental sexual phase of experimenting with relationships. Such an 'all or nothing' approach left no room for the kind of 'growth ethic' advocated by Roger Burggraeve in his article 'Meaningful living and action: an ethical and education–pastoral model in Christian perspective', in *Louvain Studies*, 1988, pp. 3–26 & 137–60. He argues for 'an interim ethics or, even stronger, "growth ethics", in so far as one approaches the period of youth as an interim phase of growth, with the stress on "growth", without losing sight of what this growth implies for provisionality and the freedom that is not yet completely developed' (p. 154).

A rigid sexual ethics also posed enormous problems in the area of birth control when couples, struggling to do their best for their families and trying to arrive at responsible decisions, felt obliged to practise forms of contraception which they had been led to believe were gravely wrong. Arriving at such a decision was a crucifying process for many people. In their heart of hearts they knew that this was the best they could do as responsible parents. Yet the only comfort traditional sexual ethics could give them was they might not be subjectively guilty of serious sin, due to their erroneous conscience or diminished freedom. The message came over loud and clear that their best was not good enough. The tragedy in all this was that what was for many a highly responsible decision arrived at only after a long process of reflective discernment still left them with a feeling of guilt and alienation from God.

A clearer appreciation of what was implicit in the accepted teaching in moral theology about conscience and also about the varying degrees of authority attached to items of moral teaching in the Roman Catholic Church could have broken the stranglehold of their dilemma. It would have enabled them to own their unformulated conviction that what they were doing was the best they could do as responsible parents and so was surely pleasing to God. God asked no more from them than that.

Such an appreciation would have opened their eyes to the possibility that Church teaching on sexual ethics is open to development, refinement and even change, in the light of our increased understanding of ourselves as sexual human persons. That would have enabled couples to appreciate that, just like themselves, the Church is only able to do the best it can in presenting what it sees to be the moral implications of the Gospel. Just as God expects no more from them than the best they can, so God expects no more – and no less – from the Church. Hence, the 'best we can do' decisions of these couples needs to allow for a similar 'best we can do' dimension in the ongoing development of the Church's sexual teaching. This means that, while listening respectfully to the Church's teaching, they need not feel unduly disturbed if, on occasion, they find this 'best we can do' teaching being questioned by responsible theologians within the Church. This will happen when these theologians have good grounds for believing that the teaching being presented by the Church authorities is not 'the best they can do' since there is available within the Church 'better' teaching than that being currently offered. When couples understand what is going on in this way, they are able to cope with the ambiguity of such a situation, appreciating that it is a natural part of the growth process within the Church. Consequently, they can feel at peace with their 'best we can do' decision, even if, on occasion, this might be at variance with current Church teaching. Moreover, their peace will further consolidated by their appreciating that their decision is 'ethically good' even though they do not have *absolute* certainty that what they are doing is 'ethically right' – though they feel pretty sure that it is.

The distinction between the 'ethical goodness' of the person in their decision-making and the 'ethical rightness' of an action can have important implications for many other problematic areas of contemporary sexual morality. In recent debates on such issues as divorce and remarriage, cohabitation, gay and lesbian relationships and so on, the language used is often vitiated by a kind of 'blame' syndrome. People who believe that sexual morality in our society is becoming 'de-moralized' in a literal sense tend to blame various groups of people who are involved in alternative sexual lifestyles. They are accused of being selfish, irresponsible, unconcerned about their children, throwing over the social order, and many other such things. They are regarded as 'blameworthy'.

However, it is possible to have a critical discussion about the various issues mentioned above without falling into the 'blame' syndrome. People living alternative sexual lifestyles may simply be questioning whether marriage, as currently lived by many people, actually achieves the human good its adherents claim for it. This is where the distinction between the 'goodness of the person' and the 'rightness of an action' can be helpful. It can enable a serious discussion to take place regarding the 'rightness' of certain forms of sexual behaviour without in any way impugning the moral good faith of those involved in such a lifestyle. Hence, it is possible to have a serious moral debate without it disintegrating into polarization. It presumes that both sides are fully committed to living authentic moral lives according to their best lights. Hence, critical observations are not heard as saying 'You are wicked in living this kind of lifestyle'. Rather their tenor is, 'Help me to understand why you are living this kind of lifestyle. When I have understood your position as fully as I can, then we will be able to discuss how this fits in with the basic fundamental values to which we are both committed.' Obviously this is a two-way process.

SEXUAL SIN AND SEXUAL SINS

As we have already seen, the fundamental criterion in a person-centred sexual ethics is what is conducive to the good of the human person, integrally and adequately considered. We have also seen that this criterion presents us with the paradox that we are more than individual instances of the species, humankind. We are unique individuals and our uniqueness permeates all the dimensions of our being – right down to our genetic make-up and even our finger-prints.

This paradox poses a problem for anyone wanting to attempt to give clear answers to particular questions regarding the morality of particular forms of human sexual behaviour. It is true that some kinds of sexual behaviour contradict what we share in common at such a fundamental level of our being that in no way could they ever be considered as being conducive to the good of the human person, integrally and adequately considered. That is because they are seriously person-injuring through being abusive or manipulative. Rape, the sexual abuse of children or their virtual slavery in the sex trade are obvious examples that come to mind. These are all destructive of persons and so in total violation of a person-centred sexual ethics. Sadly, it is not difficult to think of other similar examples of serious violation of the person. Nevertheless, sometimes our answers to specific practical questions in the field of sexual ethics can do no more than say what is valid as a general rule. Such a general answer is the best that we can offer because of the uniqueness of the particular individual, arising out of such things as his or her personal story, the stage of personal or sexual development he or she is at, and so on. Hence, a general answer might need considerable modification in some particular instances.

I would like to conclude this chapter with an example of how, using the approach outlined above, the discussion of particular questions in sexual ethics might proceed. The example I have chosen is casual and uncommitted sex.

IS IT RIGHT TO ENGAGE IN CASUAL AND UNCOMMITTED SEX?

Casual and uncommitted sex seems to be taken for granted by many young people in society today. This is certainly the assumption of many media presentations of their contemporary lifestyle. The assumption underlying this lifestyle is that there is nothing wrong with young people enjoying each other sexually, especially when they take contraceptive precautions to avoid an unwanted pregnancy. After all, life is to be enjoyed, especially when you are young. What is wrong with young people enjoying themselves in this way, provided no one gets hurt? Translated into the ethical language I have been using, the question posed by the lifestyle of many young people is: Is it right to engage in casual, uncommitted sex?

I believe that a person-centred sexual ethic gives a 'No, but . . . ' answer to that question.

No . . .

. . . because it sells us short as relational beings, capable of interpersonal love. In that sense, it is dehumanizing since it is living well below our human potential. It also fails to do justice to us as bodily persons since it involves two persons using each other's bodies for individual pleasure without interest in and concern for the profound body-person each of them is. In that sense, it could almost be described as sexual abuse. It is abusing the gift of each other's sexuality by trivializing it. Casual sex fails to respect human sexuality's capacity for intimate and joyful personal encounter at a profound level of our being, an encounter which is impossible outside of a context of mutual trust which needs to be built up gradually as two persons come to know each other at an increasingly intimate level. The case for casual sex is sometimes argued on the grounds that it is a fun thing to do. However, as Gareth Moore points out, casual sex misses out on the real fun of sex by reducing it to purely individualistic pleasure. Fun sex, in the fuller sense, involves the much deeper and more satisfying joys which are to be found in the deeply pleasurable sexual exchange of mutual love and personal commitment. Joy – probably a better word than fun – is but part of the wider coalition of profound human feelings which makes up the rich experience of a human relationship in which a couple have the security of knowing they can trust each other unreservedly. Such a relationship really is fun – but its riches are not exhausted by its fun dimension.

The 'No' of my answer applies equally to uncommitted sexual exchanges between gays or lesbians. Sometimes 'cruising' is presented as being as natural for gay men as breathing. It is portrayed as simply part of what it means to be gay. I do not find that claim supported by gay and lesbian theologians who are arguing that there is but one sexual ethics for all, regardless of sexual orientation. 'Cruising' or other forms of trivial and uncommitted gay sex would seem to be dehumanizing for precisely the same kind of reasons I have outlined above.

. . . but . . .

. . . a sexual ethics for today needs to listen to what is going on among young people. Many feel so alienated from the world of so-called responsible adults that they are trying to find some sense of identity in their youth culture. And casual sex is part of that youth culture. A thundering 'No' against casual sex is likely to be totally ineffective since it is looking at just one symptom of a much deeper and far-reaching malaise. Moreover, it is likely to be heard as coming from the very source of their alienation, an adult world which has forfeited their respect by its apparent lack of idealism. It seems to have sold its soul to individualism and supports policies which leave many young people without any real hope for the future. Young people are unlikely to listen to adults telling them that casual sex is dehumanizing when, in fact, it is the very society which is taken for granted by these same adults which young people experience as utterly dehumanizing. No doubt this was one of the things the Catholic bishops of England and Wales had in mind in their 1996 statement *The Common Good and the Catholic Church's Social Teaching* when they wrote:

> Those who advocate unlimited free-market capitalism and at the same time lament the decline in public and private morality, to which the encouragement of selfishness is a prime contributing factor, must ask themselves whether the messages they are sending are in fact mutually contradictory. (n. 80)

An editorial in *The Tablet* made a similar comment: 'No manipulation of the curriculum can coerce children into believing in Christian sexual ethics and traditional patterns of family life, if those values are not shared by their teachers, parents and national role models, and are contradicted by everything they see and hear in the mass media' (3 November 1996, p. 1431).

This book argues for a person-centred sexual ethics. That will only make sense and be feasible in the context of a society which is committed to a person-centred morality right across the board. Perhaps the trivial sex found among young people is the hurting edge of a malaise which is affecting society as a whole. I am not suggesting that casual, uncommitted sex is right for young people today. I am simply trying to understand why they are drawn to it. No doubt, some casual sex is linked to the experimental phase of adolescence, as Burggraeve has pointed out. However, much of it might actually constitute a veiled challenge to the rest of us. Perhaps the alienation of young people, symbolized by their finding comfort in casual sex, challenges the adult world to reconstruct society and our world in such a way that the dignity of human persons and their rights and obligations as individuals and social beings are the fundamental criteria against which everything else is assessed. Our human sexuality is an essential dimension of our capacity for connectedness. A society which creates unconnectedness and division does not offer a very convincing context for credible education in a positive sexual ethics.

I believe that a person-centred sexual ethics would answer many burning questions of sexual ethics (e.g. pre-marital sex, cohabitation, and so forth) with a similar kind of 'No, but . . . ' answer. The 'No' part of the answer would be saying that, as a general rule, such behaviour or such a lifestyle can hardly be regarded as conducive to the good of the human person, integrally and adequately considered. And the reasons offered for this judgement would be drawn from the basic values outlined earlier in Chapter Six. However, the 'but . . . ' part of the answer is needed to make allowance for the fact that individual moral agents are not all proceeding from the same starting-point. As noted in our exploration of structural sin, their starting-points may be vastly different. This can be due to a variety of forms of structural injustice which may seriously reduce the options open to them. It can also be due to their personal woundedness resulting from devastating negative experiences endured in earlier chapters of their life-story. As mentioned at the end of the previous chapter in my article 'Moral theology in the parish', in *Priests and People*, 1994, pp. 367–72, I used the parable of the wheat and darnel to illustrate this important facet of our moral life. I noted that the owner of the field has faith in the healthy growth of his wheat, despite all the darnel mixed in with it, and that he wants to protect his wheat from the misguided zeal of his servants intent on dragging up the darnel, regardless of the terrible harm this might do to the wheat. Sometimes moral zealots can act very destructively because they are oblivious to the fact that 'what might look like a puny and undeveloped plant might, in fact, be a miracle of growth, given the adverse conditions under which it has had to struggle' (p. 371).

I would suspect that many answers to questions about the rightness or wrongness of specific ways of acting in the sexual field should take this 'Yes, but . . . ' or 'No, but . . . ' form. The 'Yes' or 'No' part of the answer enables us to be clear as to whether or not, as a general rule, this particular form of behaviour is conducive to the good of the human person, integrally and adequately considered. This can also help to show that a contemporary person-centred sexual ethics is still substantially in continuity with the core teaching most of us were brought up with, while at the same time nuancing this teaching in ways which can radically transform the way it applies the good news of the Gospel to our everyday lives.

8

LIVING POSITIVELY IN A TIME OF AIDS

LIVING POSITIVELY WITH AIDS: A LESSON FROM UGANDA

The subtitle of this book is *Moral Theology and the Challenge of AIDS.* Having listened to the challenge of the AIDS pandemic in Chapter One, we have been exploring how Christian sexual ethics should respond. These closing two chapters bring us back to where we began, the AIDS pandemic and its impact on developing countries. This chapter will look at some of the practical implications of 'living positively with AIDS' and will examine some good and some questionable Church practice. The final chapter situates the AIDS pandemic in a global frame and suggests that responding to the challenge of 'living positively with AIDS' could actually be a time of grace for our world.

I first heard the expression 'living positively with AIDS' from the lips of Noerine Kaleeba, a Ugandan woman whom I was privileged to meet in Kampala. She is an extraordinary person. Her personal story is a living example of the meaning of 'living positively with AIDS'.

Noerine was more fortunate than many Ugandan women in that she had a good education. This led to her becoming a physiotherapist in the major hospital in Kampala. Her husband, Chris, worked in Adult Education and eventually got a scholarship to do a PhD at Hull University. He came to England in 1985. This was right in the middle of Uganda's second civil war in 10 years. During the winter of 1985 Noerine and her four daughters spent 3 days hidden in a cellar without food and water, hiding from Obote's fleeing soldiers who were killing and raping as they left. On 6 June 1986 Noerine got news that Chris was seriously ill in hospital in Hull. She was told he had AIDS.

At that time, she knew little about AIDS, connecting it with white homosexual men in San Francisco, though there had been rumours of a similar condition in the Ugandan border region of Rakai. Naturally, Noerine told her family, friends, neighbours and work colleagues about Chris's illness. She thought nothing of letting them know he had AIDS.

She flew to England and found Chris was desperately ill. The doctors counselled Noerine to have an HIV test herself. This proved negative but they warned her that this did not guarantee she was not infected with HIV. She would need to have another test at a later stage. For the sake of her daughters, Noerine had to leave Chris in September and return home. When she got back to Uganda, she found that nearly everyone began to shun her and her daughters. Due to ignorance, they thought that AIDS was infectious in a similar way to measles. This was a very difficult and isolating time for Noerine, especially with the additional strain of her being separated from Chris in his illness. When Chris's health showed some signs of improvement, he was able to return to Uganda in October. However, he soon had to go into hospital in Kampala. There, to Noerine's horror, the nurses would not even enter his room and she herself had to do all the nursing, even quite technical medical procedures. As well as shunning her, people were just waiting for Noerine herself to show signs of AIDS and start dying. The only support that Noerine and Chris got at this time was from a little group of people whose lives had also been affected by AIDS. In fact, twelve of them actually had AIDS themselves.

Eventually Chris died from AIDS-related meningitis. Noerine was totally devastated by his death, by the terrible pain in which he died and by the way she and her daughters had been treated. To make matters worse, although Chris had made a will, it was not sufficiently specific to override local custom. Consequently, in accordance with the patriarchal traditions of their culture, the house in which Noerine and her daughters were living and the bit of land that went with it did not go to her and her children but to her husband's brother. Ironically, it was only much later that Noerine discovered that Chris had probably been infected with HIV due to a blood transfusion (8 units) he had received from his brother after he had been knocked down by a bus in 1983. That brother died of AIDS the year after Chris.

Noerine believes that one of the gifts God has given her is a positive approach to life. If something is wrong and can be changed, she must do whatever she can to make things better. What she experienced in the course of Chris's illness and death convinced her that there was a great deal wrong in Uganda with regard to the AIDS scene:

- the medical care for people with AIDS was appalling;
- ignorance about AIDS was causing people living with AIDS, along with their children, to be shunned by everyone;
- the cultural subordination of women was creating a whole host of problems and these were either contributing to the spread of AIDS or were making it even more difficult for women whose husbands were infected;
- parents with AIDS were fearful about what could happen to their children when they died.

Noerine got together the sixteen people who had formed the little support group which had been so helpful to Chris and herself. They decided to try to do something practical to improve things at all these different levels. From this small beginning TASO (The AIDS Support Organization) was born. By 1994 when I visited Uganda, it was having a major impact on the AIDS scene in Kampala and many other parts of the country and was being seen as a model for other countries to follow.

Initially TASO concentrated on information-giving and counselling. The only messages people were receiving were 'AIDS kills' and 'Love faithfully and beat AIDS'. Neither of these slogans offered any hope to people who were already HIV positive. Noerine believed that they needed something more to empower them to live their lives positively. Counselling and good medical care were both needed. But factors which affected the whole family also had to be faced. So there was a need for a more holistically directed approach, including tackling the issue of behaviour change. TASO gradually developed a whole system of health workers, local clinics and trained specialist nurses to work with people with AIDS. To combat ignorance about HIV/AIDS they trained local community workers and established a comprehensive network of them in different parts of Uganda. They also established a body of trained counsellors. These were in great demand since it is not easy for a young person to discover that he or she will die soon, and even harder if they have a young family. To tackle the problem of women left without home or land they developed a whole series of income-generating projects for widows and orphans to help them be self-supporting. They also formed women's support groups to try to change the abuse of women in their culture. Linked to this they began working with a group of women lawyers who were trying to make the law more respectful of women and who were promoting the making of wills which would safeguard the rights of women when their husbands died. And finally, they got funding to pay the school fees for AIDS orphans to enable them to have a better chance in life.

When I visited TASO in 1994 they were supporting 370 orphans over an 8-year schooling programme. Sadly, they had a further 15,000 orphans on their books whom they had assessed as needing help. By 1994 TASO had 250 paid staff and its budget, mainly from overseas relief agencies, was $1.5 million per year. It had also trained 1,800 community volunteers as AIDS counsellors in the villages. Their paid workers operated in 7 centres across Uganda, all at important points along the TransAfrican Highway, and their outreach programmes covered a 40 km radius around each centre. At that time they had decided that they could not expand any further and so their priority was changing to a broadening of their educational capacity so that they could help other new groups which are springing up. Tragically, the majority of the original sixteen founding members of TASO have already died of AIDS.

Noerine has written up her personal experience in a very moving little book entitled *We Miss You All* (Harare, Zimbabwe, Women & AIDS Support Network, 1991). Her inspiring but very down-to-earth understanding of what it means to 'live positively with AIDS' comes out clearly in the following passage:

> **Living positively with AIDS**. The public health messages were saying 'Beware of AIDS. AIDS kills', 'You catch it and you are as good as dead'. There were no messages for those people who were already infected. What was implied was that people who were already infected should die and get it over. People with HIV and AIDS were seen as dying. We adopted the slogan of 'Living positively with AIDS' in direct defiance of that perception. We emphasised *living* rather than *dying* with AIDS. For us it was the quality rather than quantity of life which was important. Once infected with a deadly virus like HIV people need to take definite steps to enhance the quality of whatever life they have left. They must develop a positive attitude to life . . .
>
> The TASO slogan is 'Living positively with AIDS' and calls on everyone in society, infected or non-infected. To the person who is infected it calls on them to live responsibly with the HIV infection in their blood, to face up to the infection as a starting point. It calls on them to recognise their responsibility to society, the responsibility to retain the amount of virus they have in their

blood, and not spread it around, by making the effort not to infect others. It also calls upon people who are infected to look after themselves better, and preserve themselves until a cure comes. It calls to people who are infected to remain actively involved in society, and in social activities within society. It also calls upon the rest of society to support people with HIV infection so that they can fulfil their obligations . . . Acceptance of people with HIV or AIDS within our community is a very important starting point for dealing with the problem. (pp. 79–80)

Noerine also mentions why she refused to have a second HIV test. She was afraid that if it showed her to be HIV negative, she would be less in solidarity with other people who were living with AIDS. That is part of how she understands 'living positively with AIDS' in her own personal life.

This lengthy account of how Noerine has been living positively with AIDS and how she has inspired so many others to follow her example might seem a strange way to conclude a book on new directions in sexual ethics! Yet I believe it is most appropriate. The whole thrust of this book has been that it is not just individual men and women infected with HIV who have to live positively with AIDS. We all have to. And I have been arguing that part of living positively with AIDS for the Christian Churches involves a renewal and enrichment of our sexual ethics in response to the challenge of HIV/AIDS.

IS THE CHURCH LIVING POSITIVELY WITH AIDS? YES, BUT . . .

Because of my limited knowledge of the situation in other Churches with regard to HIV/AIDS, my answer will refer mainly, though not exclusively, to the Roman Catholic Church. Following the 'Yes, but . . . ' or 'No, but . . . ' style of answer adopted in the previous chapter, I would suggest that the answer in this case should be 'Yes, but . . . ', even though the 'but . . . ' is a large one!

I say 'Yes, but . . . ' rather than 'No, but . . . ' because my experience on the CAFOD AIDS committee has opened my eyes to the way so many Christians, right across the world, have responded extremely positively to the HIV/AIDS tragedy. In many of the developing countries, it is the Christian Churches who have led the way with immense heroism and generosity in HIV/AIDS work in all its different facets, hospital-based medical care, home care, educational work, counselling, caring for orphans, specialized work with young people, creating viable alternatives for women forced into prostitution, and so forth. The way CAFOD, for instance, has responded so creatively to the AIDS pandemic is indicative of a similar response among many other development agencies. A very moving and informative account of some magnificent AIDS projects linked together through the World Council of Church's process, *Women and Health and the Challenge of HIV/AIDS*, is found in Gillian Paterson, *Love in a Time of AIDS: Women, Health and the Challenge of HIV* (Geneva, WCC Publications and New York, Orbis, 1996).

I know from personal experience that much of the funding channelled through the CAFOD AIDS department has gone to projects which seem to be doing effective work in the following areas:

- education for AIDS prevention by raising awareness and encouraging behaviour change;
- preventative health care (testing the blood supply, clean needles, etc.);
- caring for the medical, physical and social needs of those living with AIDS;
- helping children who have become orphans through AIDS.

Because of their awareness of the 'feminization of poverty' dimension, CAFOD are always careful to examine whether projects take this into account. They know from experience that some local projects could actually be prejudicial to the interests and well-being of women. Moreover, CAFOD's involvement has always been based on listening to and supporting local people in the field. It has also been self-critical, always ready to learn from mistakes.

What about my large 'but . . . ' attached to my answering, 'Yes, the Church is living positively with AIDS'? What does that large 'but . . . ' refer to?

It refers to the many instances where, sadly, the Churches seem to be part of the problem rather than part of the solution. That this is beginning to be recognized comes out in the interesting phenomenon that some of the CAFOD AIDS staff are increasingly being asked to help priests, religious and seminarians with issues related to sexual development and attitudes in their own lives. Tragically, many priests and male religious still believe in the inferior status of women as much as anyone else and this shows itself in the way they treat women, even women religious. Moreover, sadly, many women religious in developing countries have internalized a belief in their own second-class status. Consequently, this aspect of CAFOD's work is a case of training the trainers since all these people should really be playing an important role in facilitating behaviour change. If the Church is to play its potentially powerful role in combating the underlying causes of the spread of HIV/AIDS in developing countries, it has first to change itself and its ministers (men and women) from being an integral part of the problem. I could offer many other reasons for my suggesting that the 'but . . . ' is a very large one. Many of these would be linked to the kind of issues dealt with in the third and fourth chapters of this book, namely, the sexual and economic subordination of women and the current teaching on gay and lesbian relationships.

However, rather than go over issues already covered earlier in the book, I would rather examine the question, 'Is the Church living positively with AIDS?', with particular reference to two specific issues not yet explored here and which crop up frequently in practice as well as in ethical discussions about HIV/AIDS. Consequently, I would like to explore the two questions: (1) Is a diocese or religious congregation living positively with AIDS if it demands the compulsory testing of candidates for the priesthood or the religious life? and (2) Is the Church living positively with AIDS when it opposes condom use as a help towards preventing HIV infection? My answer will be 'No' to each question.

1. Is a diocese or religious congregation living positively with AIDS if it demands the compulsory HIV testing of candidates for the priesthood or the religious life?

The question of compulsory testing is usually posed as an ethical dilemma focused on the values of personal freedom and the right to privacy. Like couples entering marriage, candidates for the priesthood and the religious life are also intending to exercise their freedom at its highest level in making a life-long commitment. Is compulsory HIV testing a violation of their freedom and their privacy?

There has been a considerable amount of writing on this point, putting forward all the points for and against such a policy. In favour of testing it is argued that such a requirement is not a violation of the candidate's freedom. After all, the candidate is making a life commitment to a particular diocese or religious congregation. Surely, it is claimed, a diocese or congregation has every right to lay down conditions for entry which they believe to have an important bearing on their ministry and mission. In a parallel instance, would it be a violation of her fiancé's freedom if a young woman insisted that he should have an HIV test before she agreed to marry him? In the case of a diocese or religious congregation, it is argued that it is legitimate for them to check out whether the health prospects of candidates are such that there is a reasonable hope that they will be able to spend an adequate number of years in active ministry or at least without being a financial burden on the limited financial resources of the diocese or congregation because of deteriorating health. These finances have, after all, been donated principally for the support of ministry and mission. Moreover, canon law would seem to allow for such a requirement.

What about the arguments against testing? Some argue that HIV testing does not provide the kind of assurance that a diocese or religious congregation is looking for in terms of future health prospects. While that might be true, it would seem to be equally true that testing provides the only level of assurance that is available, however inadequate it may be. However, there are other problems involved in testing. The HIV test can give a wrong result. Also testing can result in excluding from the priesthood or religious life people who might still have many years of healthy, active life before them, despite their being HIV positive. The freedom dimension is also linked to the right to privacy. Obligatory testing of all candidates is undoubtedly an intrusion into a person's privacy. This would need to be justified by some compensating major positive gain to the common good. That needs to be proved rather than assumed, especially in view of the fact that anyone who has been tested, regardless of the test, often becomes the object of discrimination on the part of insurance companies and other financial institutions. Since such discrimination is the result of the testing policy of the diocese or religious congregation, it could be argued that the diocese or congregation is obliged to accept at least some responsibility for any financial loss incurred by a prospective candidate as a result of the ensuing discrimination.

Very deliberately I posed the initial question about compulsory testing not in terms of respect for freedom and privacy but in terms of living positively with AIDS. I have repeatedly insisted in this book that we are living in a 'time of AIDS'. Many would argue that in this 'time of AIDS', there is a special moral imperative (even a 'call from God') on dioceses and religious congregations to stand positively with those who are living with HIV/AIDS. At the very least, this would mean doing nothing that might seem to lend support to the tendency of many in society to marginalize people living with HIV/AIDS or which might increase the negative self-image and sense of alienation such marginalization can cause. In fact, it could even be argued that the acceptance within the diocesan priesthood or in a religious congregation of people with HIV/AIDS might provide a very powerful counter-witness to those who look on HIV/AIDS as only affecting 'people out there' and not really 'any of our concern', or who impose a stigma on anyone living with HIV/AIDS. Belief in the Church as a sign and instrument of the unity of the human family implies living in solidarity with people living with HIV/AIDS. Theologically, this has been captured in the expression, 'the Church has AIDS'. The presence of people living with HIV/AIDS in the priesthood and the religious life might help to bring home that important truth. At a meeting of Asian theologians on HIV/AIDS which I attended in Bangkok, I recorded in my diary that one of the theologians present, himself a religious, 'said that he dreamt of the day when every religious congregation would have HIV+ members who would be fully accepted and valued among them as religious. He believed that the congregations would be all the healthier for this.'

This last point, that in this 'time of AIDS' compulsory HIV testing for future priests and religious would give a counter-witness to the Gospel values we believe in clinches the argument for me. Therefore, I believe that 'living positively with AIDS' excludes such compulsory testing.

2. Is the Church living positively with AIDS when it opposes using condoms as a help towards preventing HIV infection?

There are two distinct issues which need to be treated quite separately here. One concerns condom use as a component in governmental HIV prevention programmes. The other concerns the use of condoms within marriage when one partner is HIV infected.

(a) Condom use as a component in governmental HIV prevention programmes

One of the health measures adopted in many countries has been to encourage non-HIV-infected people to use condoms if they are going to have sex with someone they cannot be absolutely sure is free of the virus. One phase of AIDS policy in the UK consisted in a massive and very expensive campaign along those lines. This policy later came in for strong criticism from the gay community on the grounds that, due to the government's unwillingness to appear supportive of gay sex, this campaign had diverted resources from where they were needed much more urgently, that is, to promote educational work among the gay community themselves since, at that point in time, they were the ones most at risk.

The Catholic Church has tended to object to this 'safer sex' educational policy and its promotion of condom use. It claims that such a campaign ignores the moral dimension of sexual activity, namely, its relational side. What is needed, it is argued, is to encourage young people to take the relational dimension of sex more seriously. Hence, the Church has refused to participate in any 'safer sex' campaigns and has limited its contribution to the 'relationship' agenda. One of the few slight modifications to this united front on the part of the Church is found in the first letter of the US Bishops' Conference on HIV/AIDS, 'The many faces of AIDS: a gospel response', issued on 11 December 1987. (The full text was published in *Origins*, 24 December 1987, pp. 481–9.) It contained the following passage:

> Because we live in a pluralistic society, we acknowledge that some will not agree with our understanding of human sexuality. We recognise that public educational programs addressed to a wide audience will reflect the fact that some people will not act as they can and should; that they will not refrain from the type of sexual or drug abuse behaviour which can transmit AIDS. In such situations educational efforts, if grounded in the broader moral vision outlined above, could include accurate information about prophylactic devices or other practices proposed by some medical experts as potential means of preventing AIDS. We are not promoting the use of prophylactics, but merely providing information that is part of the factual picture. Such a factual presentation should indicate that abstinence outside of marriage and fidelity within marriage as well as the avoidance of intravenous drug abuse are the only morally correct and medically sure ways to prevent the spread of AIDS. So-called safe sex practices are at best only partially effective. They do not take into account either the real values that are at stake or the fundamental good of the human person. (p. 486)

This letter was issued by the Administrative Board of the US Bishops' Conference without being cleared by the Conference as a whole. When it appeared it provoked an outcry, not least among some of the bishops themselves, most notably Cardinal O'Connor of New York. In the light of this negative reaction, although this pastoral letter was never officially withdrawn, a replacement letter was put together. Entitled

'Called to compassion and responsibility: a response to the HIV/AIDS crisis', it appeared on 9 November 1989. It was issued in the name of the whole Bishops' Conference and gave no hint of toleration towards any preventive health policy involving the promotion or distribution of condoms. It simply asserted that 'advocating this approach means in effect promoting behaviour which is morally unacceptable'. Between the two letters and as a comment on the first letter, Cardinal Ratzinger had written to the papal nuncio, Archbishop Laghi, stating the real cause of the AIDS problem was 'the permissiveness which, in the area of sex as in that related to other abuses, corrodes the moral fibre of the people' (quoted in Richard L. Smith, *Aids, Gays and the American Catholic Church*, p. 66).

Another slight breach in the Catholic Church's united front opposing promotion of the use of condoms in HIV educational programmes was detected by some critics in the HIV/AIDS educational pack produced for schools by the Archdiocese of Edinburgh. This carried an *imprimatur* from the Archdiocese. According to a report in the *Guardian* (11 November 1995) the Congregation for the Doctrine of the Faith (CDF) 'criticised the pack for advocating the use of condoms for people who are HIV positive'. The actual wording found in the pack itself read:

> Medically it has been shown that condoms do reduce the risk of infection but they are not 100% safe, and should not be seen as the answer to the problem. They do not make for safe sex. In marriage where one or both partners are HIV-positive, and the couple wish to continue to express their love sexually, they have a right and duty to use protection.

The CDF asked for the *imprimatur* to be withdrawn and for Catholic educational institutions to cease using the pack (cf. *Briefing*, 16 November 1995, p. 39).

A similar opposition to the promotion and use of condoms as a health measure has been characteristic of most bishops' conferences in developing countries too. As a result, many have publicly opposed any Government HIV/AIDS campaigns involving the promotion of condom-use for the purposes of 'safer sex'.

More recently in 1996 the Social Commission of the French bishops' conference produced a 235-page symposium on AIDS entitled *SIDA: La société en question* (Paris, Bayard Editions/Centurion). The press coverage gave the impression that this constituted a major defence of the use of the condom in public health campaigns to prevent HIV transmission. In fact, the text is highly critical of such 'safer sex' campaigns and argues that at a public level they can do more harm than good. However, in a personal contribution to the symposium the president of the Social Commission, Bishop Albert Rouet, concedes that the use of condoms is 'understandable in the case of people for whom sexual activity is already an integral part of their lives and there is serious risk of their being infected by the virus' (p. 194, n. 49). However, he immediately adds that 'this course of action does not help to educate a person towards sexual maturity'. The general tone of the symposium reflects a conviction that the HIV/AIDS pandemic is an indication that there is something badly wrong in society. It argues that this underlying evil urgently needs to be tackled.

Although this document was less open to condom use than was suggested by press reports, it provided reporters with the opportunity of discovering that a number of bishops had independently adopted a similar line to Bishop Rouet. For instance, it was reported in *The Tablet* (24 February 1996, p. 272) that a 'less than absolute prohibition' stance had been taken by Cardinals Lustiger, Simonis and Eyt and the late Cardinals Decourtray and Coffy, as well as by Archbishop Aguilar and Bishops Bonfils and Cornet. Of particular interest is the statement of Bishop Alanis: 'If, with the use of the condom, we can save the harmony of the conjugal union, I believe that can be admissible.' Bishop Victor Guazzelli's comment to *The Tablet* is particularly noteworthy: 'It seems to me that if people are set on intercourse they at least have the obligation of not passing on disease and death, even if the only means possible to them is the use of the condom. This seems to be common sense.' I suspect many readers will say 'Amen' to that! After all, though there may be disagreements about how sexual loving is intended by God to be 'life-giving', there is surely no disagreement that God certainly did not intend it to be 'death-dealing'.

A number of points need to be made in this connection.

First of all, the anti-condom approach seems to ignore the fact that concern for bodily health is actually a moral issue. A government health authority would be failing in its duty if it did not do everything it could to safeguard and promote the health of its citizens. Hence, it needs to be recognized that in encouraging citizens to act in a way which offers less of a health risk a government is encouraging its citizens to behave more ethically. To oppose a government following this course of action would seem to be tantamount to obstructing a government in carrying out its moral obligations towards its citizens.

Some bishops have objected that to promote the use of condoms for 'safer sex' is to mislead people. The use of a condom does not guarantee there will be no risk of infection. Hence, a pro-condom campaign can give people a false sense of security. This objection is legitimate to the extent that it is engaging the issue precisely on health grounds. These bishops are claiming that, precisely as a health measure, this is not a good policy. A similar claim was made in a letter to *The Tablet* (25 November 1995, pp. 1508–9) by Dr Michael Jarmulowicz of the Guild of Catholic Doctors. The problem, however, is that this objection does not seem to be valid in the light of the best scientific evidence currently available. In a subsequent letter this is pointed out by Dr Michael Abbott, a consultant genito-urinary physician caring for people living with HIV/AIDS:

> Two kinds of data (i.e. *in vitro* and *in vivo*) have been collected on the relationship between barrier methods of contraception and sexually transmitted diseases. The *in vitro* data generally show that high-quality latex condoms are impermeable to the passage of HIV and other organisms. As regard *in vivo* studies, what is clear is that consistent condom use confers substantial protection against HIV transmission but that inconsistent use carries considerable risk of HIV infection. (*The Tablet*, 9 December 1995, p. 1579)

Dr Abbott's point is corroborated by the Jesuit physician, Dr Jon Fuller, who is Assistant Director in the Clinical AIDS Programme at Boston City Hospital and Assistant Clinical Professor of Medicine at Boston University School of Medicine. Dr Fuller, too, is immersed in working with people living with the virus. In his *HIV/AIDS: An Overview*, (Chicago, National Conference of Priests, 1995), he writes:

> For those who choose to engage in high risk behaviours despite all warnings, the routine use of latex condoms can decrease the risk of acquiring HIV. There is no doubt that a number of factors can contribute to the failure rate of condoms, including improper timing in the use or improper technique in their application . . . Due to these multiple potential sources of error, the pregnancy rate for condoms has often been quoted as quite high, often in the neighbourhood of 10–15%. However, these statistics may represent the intermittent employment of condoms by inexperienced users. Studies with couples who use condoms correctly all the time have reported pregnancy rates as low as 2%. More recent data from three studies evaluating the use of condoms to prevent HIV transmission from one infected member of a stable sexual relationship to the individual's uninfected partner suggest that

consistent and correct use of latex condoms can significantly reduce the risk of acquiring HIV in this situation.

One observational study followed 245 HIV-discordant hetero-sexual couples (in which one member is HIV-infected and the other is not) for a median of 22 months; in all, the only risk for the uninfected member to become HIV-infected was intercourse with his or her infected partner. In retrospect, half of the group had used condoms 100% of the time, the other half had used them intermittently. As compared with 12 documented infections in the group using condoms intermittently, no infections were observed among those who used them consistently despite an estimated 15,000 episodes of intercourse.

In another study of 282 Greek prostitutes, no infections occurred over an observation period of two years among a group who had increased its use of condoms from 66% to 97% of the time. This change was also accompanied by a decrease in the frequency of syphilis from 17% to 3%, and in gonococcal infection from 14% to 0%.

A third study compared transmission rates from infected haemophiliacs to their sexual partners. Among 31 couples, 14 always used condoms, and 17 used them occasionally or not at all. Over an observation period of two years, there were 3 sero-conversions in the intermittent use group (a 17% transmission rate), compared with no infections in the consistent use group. (pp. 29–30)

Moreover, in his 1996 Distinguished Jesuit Lecture, 'AIDS Prevention and the Catholic Moral Tradition', at St Louis University Health Sciences Center, Dr Fuller mentions some new population-based data from Uganda and Thailand which also seem to indicate that condom-use can have a significant impact on HIV prevention. For instance, the Thai government's *100% Condom Campaign* increased the use of condoms by commercial sex workers from 50 per cent to more than 94 per cent in the space of four years. Dr Fuller notes that this 'was accompanied by a reduction in sexually transmitted diseases – taken to be a surrogate marker for new HIV infections – from 6.5 per 1,000 to 1.64 per 1,000 ('AIDS prevention: a challenge to the Catholic moral tradition', in *America*, 28 December 1996, pp. 13–20, at p. 18). In a country where HIV infection is running at 2 per cent of the population and where many married men frequent commercial sex workers, it is estimated that the success of the government's campaign has had a notable impact as a HIV prevention measure.

Dr Fuller accepts the the the significance of the above evidence for government programmes which include condom-use as one component of
their overall strategy. He believes that the studies cited 'demonstrate
that these approaches can be part of the solution, that in real life
situations they have significantly prevented HIV transmission and have
saved many lives'. However, he repeats his warning that 'condoms
cannot be taken as an absolute guarantee against infection during
intercourse'. He states very clearly that 'condoms cannot make unsafe
sex safe; they only make it less unsafe'. Nevertheless, he still insists
that 'for those individuals who choose to engage in high risk activities,
condoms can reduce the risk'.

In the light of this evidence, therefore, it would seem highly responsible for a government, as a part of its HIV educational programme,
to encourage very strongly the use of condoms by those who, despite
all warnings, insist on engaging in high-risk activities. The same would
be true for individual doctors, including Catholic doctors. I fully agree
with Dr Abbott's judgement when he writes:

> I, and the vast majority of Catholic doctors I know, would have no
> hesitation whatsoever in recommending the use of condoms if a
> patient with HIV infection or any other sexually transmissible
> infection (whatever their marital status or sexual orientation)
> intended to have sexual relations with another person. (*The Tablet*,
> 9 December 1995, p. 1579)

It might be objected that the Church is in the business of moral
education, not health education. Though there is some truth in that
objection, it can also be dangerously misleading. Concern for health is
a moral issue. It certainly loomed large in the ministry of Jesus. In fact,
he seems to have placed health-care above the dictates of religious
observance in some of his confrontations with the Pharisees. In the
light of the evidence quoted by Dr Fuller regarding the health benefits
of condom-use for prostitutes, I cannot help thinking that Jesus's angry
reaction to the Pharisees when they objected to some of his cures on
the Sabbath would have been equally in place when some misguided
Filipino Church officials forced the Bethany Growth House drop-in
centre for prostitutes to stop instructing their clients about the use of
condoms (cf. *AIDS in the Philippines: A Situation Analysis*, JIC, 1994, p. 74).

Spokespersons for the Catholic Church often argue, with some
justification, that 'safer sex' education is short-sighted and sells health
concerns short. The only behaviour-change that will really prevent the
spread of the AIDS virus is the observance of strict moral standards

in the field of sexual ethics – 'no sex before marriage', 'no sex outside marriage' and 'no sex between same-sex couples'. However, the problem with this position is that the Church seems to be asking the state to present the Church's *ethical* teaching under the guise of *health* teaching. Obviously, the Church has every right to offer its ethical vision of good human relationships to the nation. It can even argue that following this vision is the road to better psychosomatic health. It is even legitimate for the Church to seek by democratic means to persuade the nation that it should embrace this kind of moral code as its agreed common morality, though here it would also need to insist that the state guarantees the freedom of those who, on conscientious grounds, cannot accept this common morality. However, what the Church cannot do is demand that the state should refrain from what it considers to be important features of health education simply because the behaviour involved runs counter to the Church's moral teaching. Such a demand would seem to be all the more unreasonable on the part of the Church when it is a case of moral teaching which does not seem to be accepted by a good proportion of the Church's membership.

It is not strictly accurate to say that the AIDS virus is being spread because of immoral behaviour. It is being spread mainly because people who have the virus are having sex with people who are not infected. That is a medically accurate reading of the situation. At this level, the only fully effective way of stopping the virus spreading is for such sexual behaviour to stop. Failing this, the next best thing is ensure that when such sexual behaviour occurs, the possibility of the virus being passed on is reduced as much as possible.

There is no way a government can step in and control all the sexual behaviour of its citizens, short of a George Orwell scenario. The permanent quarantining of all HIV positive persons would be making those infected the scapegoat for society's problem. It would be ignoring the fact that, in very many cases, the spread of the virus is due to the irresponsible behaviour of non-infected people. It is likely that a strict quarantine policy would only be possible in a highly totalitarian society. Yet it is remarkable that the quarantine policy followed in Cuba, contrary to the horror stories circulated about it, was conducted in an increasingly humane fashion. It also seems to have been extremely successful as a method of HIV prevention in the country. An interesting account of this policy has been written up by Nancy Scheper-Hughes, 'AIDS and the social body', in *Social Science and Medicine*, 1994, pp. 991–1003. As we seen already, those who are particularly at risk through such irresponsible behaviour are prostitutes and other young people, even children, who are victims of the sex industry. Almost certainly they would be targeted as the identifiable groups who would be made the scapegoats in any quarantine policy.

Probably the best a government can do in a democratic society is to launch an educational drive to encourage behaviour change. According to what we have considered already, this should have two components to it from a health point of view.

The first should be aimed at making people who know they are HIV positive more aware of their responsibility not to pass the virus on to others. It would point out that the most effective way to do this is to refrain from any sexual activity which would put others at risk. Failing that – and, in the case of a married couple when one is infected, that scenario need not imply anything morally questionable – the next best option is to make sexual activity as safe as possible through the use of a condom.

The second component should be directed at those who are uninfected by the virus. It should be aimed at making them more aware of their responsibility to take care of their own health. Hence, it will need to provide accurate information about how the virus is transmitted and what steps can be taken to prevent this transmission. Clearly, discussion of condom-use and the provision of accurate information about its effectiveness in preventing transmission of the virus will be part of this educational package.

However, such a policy should not be limited to purely health considerations. The moral climate of a country is very much the concern of a government, even though responsibility for this climate is shared by the whole community and, in a particular way, by the Churches and other religious bodies. Education in a positive sexual ethic should be a major concern of any government striving to prevent the spread of HIV infection. The argument of this book is that a Christian sexual ethics should be positive, joyful, life-loving, attractive and celebratory of our sexuality. If the Churches are willing to listen to and sympathize with the government's concern for all dimensions of a health education programme, there is more likelihood that the government will be supportive of personal rela- tionship educational programmes which are based on such a positive sexual ethic.

(b) The use of condoms within marriage when one partner is HIV infected

When one partner is HIV positive or has advanced to full-blown AIDS, something new enters into their relationship which affects them both. Given the nature of HIV/AIDS, the infected partner might well feel an extra need for that love and reassurance which can be expressed so deeply in marital intimacy. And the other partner, if sensitive to that need, might well be all the more anxious to respond fully to that need. Since they have both made that high-level exercise of their freedom in giving themselves to each other in their marriage commitment, they believe that that commitment must be honoured by making love, especially now in this 'time of AIDS' in their lives. If their love-making is, as Vatican II teaches, a channel of God's love for each of them, they might well feel the need for it all the more at this crucial time.

However, they also recognize that safeguarding the health of the non-infected partner is a moral concern for both of them, if they are truly to respect each other as human persons. This serious moral obligation will take on an additional gravity if they have children who are likely to end up dependent on the care of the non-infected parent. A morality based on the dignity of the human person will have no difficulty in recognizing that such a couple may, and even should, use a condom if their love-making involves sexual intercourse. In doing so, they are being true to their dignity as human persons. They are, therefore, doing what is God's will for them.

Bob Vitillo recounts a very telling incident in this connection:

> In one workshop which I was conducting in the Philippines, a religious sister stated that HIV-infected persons would simply stop having sexual relations if they really 'loved' their partners. One lay woman in the group quickly added the correction: 'You do not understand what married love involves, Sister. If my husband were infected with HIV, I would need to continue my sexual relationship with him in order to express the fullness of my love for him and to receive strength and comfort from him on the long road ahead of us.' (unpublished address to National Catholic AIDS Ministry Conference, Chicago, 25 July 1994, p. 10)

Another HIV/AIDS scenario might be one in which the relationship between the couple is oppressive of the wife's freedom and far from the high level of equality and mutuality present in the above story. If it is the husband who is HIV positive in this case and if he demands intercourse as his right from his wife, sexual ethics must make it crystal-clear that this is not his 'right'. He has no right to endanger the health of his wife in this way. She has every right to refuse him, unless he is prepared to take adequate precautions. Obviously, in such a situation, it may be very difficult, even dangerous, for a wife to refuse her husband. To do so could put her at risk in a different way, as a result of her husband's violence towards here. A scenario like this presents a pastoral challenge to the Church on a number of fronts:

- The Church's earlier understanding implicitly legitimated this kind of behaviour and attitude on the part of a husband. Today we recognize that this violates the Church's own criterion of the dignity of the human person. Hence, every effort needs to be made to disabuse both husbands and wives of this earlier understanding and so reduce the harm it is still causing, especially to women, within marriage.
- The criterion of the dignity of the human person means that, if a wife feels she has to agree to sex in the kind of scenario envisaged above, any Church official who told her that it would better if her husband did not use a condom would be perpetrating a serious injustice against her.
- As long as a lower-level interpretation of marriage is still in practical operation, it would seem that an important dimension of the Church's work of marriage preparation and continuing support for couples would be in the area of assertiveness-training for wives. This might be more necessary in some cultures than in others.

Epilogue

A TIME OF AIDS – A TIME OF GRACE?

A 'TIME OF AIDS'

Throughout this book I have often mentioned that we are living in a 'time of AIDS'. The word 'time' in that expression is not used in a purely chronological sense (e.g. I am writing these words at 5.15 p.m. on 23 Oct 1996). Rather, it is used in a more theological sense, that is, in the sense of a *kairos* or 'defining moment', a moment of opportunity which might never return. In other words, a moment in time can be called 'theological' when what we are currently experiencing in life seems to hold a clear and compelling call from God to us. I would even dare to suggest that such a time presents us with a 'creation' moment, an invitation to set in motion another 'big bang'. Such would be the case when the negativity underlying what is happening in life is revealed so starkly that it elicits from us the natural reaction, 'This must not be allowed to continue. This is in contradiction to what life is meant to be all about.' Edward Schillebeeckx calls such a moment a 'contrast experience', a time of hearing God's voice calling to us through the cries of human suffering (cf. *God, the Future of Man*, London, Sheed & Ward, 1969, pp. 149–61). What is happening is a clear contrast to how God wants us to live. It is as though the negativity we are facing embodies the powers of darkness and out of this darkness we hear the voice of God crying out, 'Let there be light!'. Since we claim, as Christians, to have had a unique historical experience of listening to God's word and of continuing the search to discern its message for today, we ought to be particularly sensitive to such a call. Vatican II reminded us of this with its insistence on the need to be attentive to 'the signs of the times'. Yet in a global determining moment God's call to conversion and action is meant for our whole human family, not just for the Church. Hence, if the Church claims to be, in the words of Vatican II, a 'sacrament or instrumental sign of intimate union with God and of the unity of all humanity' (*Constitution on the Church*, n. 1), it cannot listen to this call on its own. The whole human family needs to listen to God's call together. It belongs to the prophetic role of the Church to play a part in enabling that to happen.

The basic premise of this book is that an awareness seems to be growing that the AIDS pandemic presents us with such a defining moment in human history. Although many who are voicing this awareness are not speaking specifically as Christians, it is also being proclaimed loud and clear by an increasing number of Christians, especially those most actively involved in the field of HIV/AIDS.

In a strange little book, *AIDS: Heresy and Prophecy: What the Virus Says* (New Delhi, Theological Research and Communication Institute, 1993), Valson Thampu comments on the fact that many people who are living positively with AIDS seem to find their experience of life deepened and intensified. In the words of Thampu they 'see this period not only in terms of impending death but also in terms of heightened life' (p. 76). He even goes so far as to refer to this time as the 'space of grace'. Not everyone involved in the AIDS scene will be happy with this kind of language. They know from tragic experience that for many others, sadly, AIDS is a totally negative and personally destructive experience, even in some cases culminating in suicide embraced as a longed-for release.

Like Thampu, I have been very struck by the fact that, paradoxically, for many people AIDS has been the occasion for their finding a new sense of meaning and purpose in their lives. In such cases expressions like Thampu's 'space of grace' and 'intensification of experience' capture very well what seems to be going on in their lives. It might be helpful to offer a few examples.

At a conference on HIV/AIDS which drew together Asian theologians from many different countries, those attending were deeply moved by the witness of a man and a woman, both living with AIDS. Though neither of them had had much formal education, their testimony played a major part in shaping the thinking of the conference. Both of them witnessed to this intensification of experience in their lives. One of them, a former taxi-driver and married man who had slept around a good deal, even went so far as to say that, compared to his life now, his life prior to AIDS was like night compared to day. They had both developed a deeper sense of self-worth and were devoting their lives to helping others affected by HIV/AIDS. They felt they had something to live for.

Nearer to home, speaking on a BBC2 programme, *The Spark*, in August 1994 in the series *Over the Edge*, Charles Irvine, a Glaswegian now working with 'Body Positive' in Manchester, spoke in very similar terms when he remarked: 'AIDS has given a lot of people a sense of purpose, a shared faith, something to live for in life – to work for others, not just self, with a sense of common purpose – to live for and even to die for.' There are some striking examples of this intensification of experience found in the book *Embracing the Chaos: Theological Responses to AIDS*, edited by James Woodward (London, SPCK, 1991). For instance, reporting on a conference held at the London Lighthouse, Stephen Pattison noted that some of those who were HIV positive in his group described their experience as being 'analogous to being converted'. His description continued: 'Suddenly life becomes both very precious and very precarious. It is important to live every second; everything from fear to hope is very vivid. It is not an exaggeration to say that some people felt they had really come to life for the first time at this fateful moment, a moment both unfair and wonderful' (p. 11). Later he went on to say: 'The people living closely with HIV/AIDS who met at the London Lighthouse (itself perhaps a sort of cathedral in this context!) were deeply alive and aware people converted to life by the threat of death' (loc. cit.).

The very moving testimony from Nigel Sheldrick which I have quoted at the end of Chapter Four is another powerful example of this intensification of experience. Some of the HIV positive women I met in Uganda were living examples of this gift of living life with deeper intensity and commitment. Similarly, I can remember three men I met on my visit to Bangkok, all HIV positive through contact with prostitutes. All three have experienced profound healing – not of the virus but of that attitude and lifestyle which led to their infection and caused them to be shunned by family and friends as a health hazard. Today, far from being a health hazard, they are helping to promote healthy living by their HIV/AIDS educational work. One of these men said to me, 'AIDS is my gift'! When I returned from Uganda, I told the people in my parish that I had brought them a gift from many of the people I had met who were living with AIDS. It was the gift of appreciating the giftedness of the present moment, the preciousness of each day and the opportunity it offers us to continue making our own unique contribution, however small, to forwarding God's Kingdom in our midst.

In the case of the people I have mentioned above, as for many others like them, the tragedy of their HIV infection seems to have presented them with a creative moment and their positive response has released new energy and light in their lives. It would be totally inaccurate to say that for them 'living positively with AIDS' is simply a matter of making the best out of a bad situation. It is much more than that. It is about beginning to live life more fully, more intensely, with greater awareness and with deeper impact on all who are touched by their lives.

A TIME OF GRACE: AIDS – A WINDOW OF OPPORTUNITY FOR OUR GLOBAL SOCIETY?

Has this 'intensification of experience' occasioned by AIDS in the lives of many individual men and women any parallel at a more global level? It seems to me that it has. Although he does not use the terminology of 'intensification of experience', it is possible to detect a global version of this phenomenon in what has been said by Richard Parker, Professor of Medical Anthropology and Human Sexuality at the State University of Rio de Janeiro. In July 1996 he presented a major paper, 'Empowerment, community mobilization and social change in the face of HIV/AIDS', at the 9th International Conference on AIDS held in Vancouver. He is very concerned that the HIV/AIDS situation is deteriorating in many ways, especially in relation to the developing world. Despite that, he is still able to view the present as a 'window of opportunity' in terms of responding to the pandemic. Parker detects a fundamental shift in our response to the HIV/AIDS pandemic and identifies three key dimensions in this shift.

The first shift is from 'individual risk' to 'social vulnerability'. The former approach stressed that specific behaviours by individuals posed the risk of HIV infection. This was soon refined into talking about 'risk groups', collections of individuals whose lifestyle was presumed to be high-risk. However, as the global pandemic progressed, this 'individual risk' model was quickly called into question, mainly because the spread of HIV infection soon went far beyond these risk groups, but also because it was creating very harmful stigma and discrimination against individuals belonging to these risk groups. Nevertheless, though not contained within these risk groups, the spread of HIV infection was not purely random. Despite the insistence of certain educational programmes that everyone was equally at risk (a 'necessary fiction', comments Parker), HIV/AIDS has never been a 'democratic epidemic'. It follows a clearly defined pattern which is structured by 'very real social, cultural, political and economic circumstances' (p. 5). For Parker, the notion of 'social vulnerability' is the key to this understanding of how HIV/AIDS infection spreads. The factors which foster its spread are 'social inequality and injustice, prejudice and discrimination, oppression, exploitation and violence' (p. 6). As a result of this clearer perception, we are now 'able to more fully comprehend the consequences, with regard to HIV infection and AIDS, of (1) the sexual stigma and discrimination so often faced by gay men or sex workers, (2) the gender power relations and gender oppression so often faced by women, and (3) the social and economic marginalization faced by the poor' (pp. 6–7). The development of this 'critical consciousness' is an important dimension in the shift in focus with regard to HIV/AIDS. It has major implications for determining effective policies and programmes for HIV prevention and control.

The second shift is from 'information/persuasion-based behaviour intervention' to 'collective empowerment and community mobilization'. An 'individual risk' approach naturally tries to promote behaviour change by giving individuals and high-risk groups sufficient information about HIV infection so that they will appreciate the risks entailed in their behaviour and change accordingly. Hence, the focus, according to this model, is on information giving and reasoned persuasion. However, this model for promoting behaviour change has not worked. As Parker says, this has been shown 'in study after study'. Hence, in line with the 'social vulnerability' model, there has been a move towards what Parker calls 'collective empowerment and community mobilization'. This is very much in line with the Paulo Freire approach based on 'conscientization'. Coming together, the socially vulnerable build up a critical perception of the 'social, cultural, political and economic forces that structure reality' and, working out of this awareness, are better able to take action against those forces which are seen to be oppressive. This model demands a whole new approach to public health with regard to vulnerable communities. While not ignoring the health care needs of individuals, its main focus is on empowering communities to respond to these needs and also to develop effective programmes of action aimed at confronting the root causes of their social vulnerability.

Parker sees the third shift to be one from 'individual-based behavioural change' to a 'global coalition for social change'. The urgent needs of individuals living with HIV/AIDS must never be neglected. However, these short-term responses must be properly integrated into much wider and long-term strategy. Since 'social vulnerability' is the key to this whole shift of approach, this long-term strategy needs to develop what Parker calls a 'global coalition' (p. 13). He explains clearly what he means by this:

> Without effecting long-term changes in the structure of society, . . . there can be no real hope of ending or even slowing the epidemic. Without overcoming the consistent denial of their basic rights and dignity, gay and bisexual men, sex workers and injecting drug users will continue to suffer the effects of the epidemic, independent of the degree of behavioural change on the part of individuals within these groups. Without transforming the unequal relations of gender power that exist in virtually every society, women around the world will continue to be preferential targets of HIV infection and will be unable to negotiate and guarantee their own safety. Without redressing the social and economic injustice that exists both within nations as well as between the developed and developing world, the poor (both in the North and in the South) will continue to suffer the major impact of an epidemic that has already become all-too-intimately linked to poverty and misery. (pp. 10–11)

Parker concludes by referring to the present time as a 'window of opportunity' (p. 12). However, he believes that a solution can be found only by our moving away from concentrating on our self-interest as individuals to a commitment to solidarity based on concern for the common good. As Richard Rorty puts it: 'moral progress can perhaps be found only in our growing capacity to overcome the oppositions that exist between our notions of "us" and "them"' (quoted in Parker, 1996, p. 14). Parker adds: 'It is in this expanding notion of "us" that the essence of human solidarity . . . can be found: by assuming the pain and suffering of others as our own, we are moved to take responsibility for the collective struggle to change it' (p. 14).

Many individuals living with HIV/AIDS experience a conversion to living more fully and with more commitment to what life is all about. Our human family is now living with HIV/AIDS. Will that experience turn out to be a conversion experience for us? I would interpret Parker as saying that it has all the potentiality for being a global conversion experience if we are prepared to be open to the critical awareness it is awakening in so many people and if we are also prepared to be enriched by being part of the global coalition for social change indicated by this critical awareness. In the Introduction to her book *AIDS in the UK: The Making of Policy, 1981–1994* (Oxford University

Press, 1996), Virginia Berridge explores various ways of understanding 'history' when looking at such a recent human phenomenon as AIDS. Though he is not a theologian, I would interpret Parker's interest in history as being more theological, using 'theological' in the same sense as I did earlier with regard to 'time'. For Parker, how we today respond to the challenge of HIV/AIDS 'will write the history of the epidemic in years to come' (p. 15). Theologically, I would suggest, our world is faced with a redemptive moment. If that is not a challenge to Christians and Christian Churches, what is?

BIBLIOGRAPHY

(1) AIDS AND DEVELOPING COUNTRIES

Bayer, Ronald, 'As the second decade of AIDS begins: an international perspective on the ethics of the epidemic', in *AIDS*, 1992, 527–32.

Bayer, Ronald, 'AIDS prevention and cultural sensitivity: Are they compatible?', in *American Journal of Public Health*, 1994, 895–8.

Bledsoe, Caroline, 'The politics of AIDS, condoms and heterosexual relations in Africa: recent evidence from the local print media', in Handwerker, W. P. (ed.), *Births and Power: Social Change and the Politics of Reproduction*, San Francisco, Westview Press, 1990, 197–223.

Campbell, Ian, *Trends and Involvement of Development NGOs in HIV/AIDS Work*, London, Salvation Army, 1994.

Cleland, John and Ferry, Benoit, *Sexual Behaviour and AIDS in the Developing World*, London, Taylor & Francis/WHO, 1995.

Durham Group, *Ethical Implications of AIDS Policies*, Durham, 1991.

Jeffrey, Paul, 'Latin America confronts AIDS', in *America*, 13 February 1993, 10–12.

Klouda, Tony, 'Responding to AIDS: Are there any appropriate development and health policies?', in *Journal of International Development*, 1995, 467–87.

Mann, Jonathan, Tarantola, Daniel J. M. and Netter, Thomas W. (eds), *AIDS in the World: A Global Report*, New York, Harvard Press, 1992.

McKenna, Neil, *On the Margins: Men Who Have Sex with Men and HIV in the Developing World*, London, Panos Institute, 1996.

Merson, M. H. 'Women and children with HIV: the global experience' (Paper to 2nd International Conference on HIV in Children and Mothers, Edinburgh, 7 Sept 1993), World Health Organization, 1993.

NAZ Project, *Report on the First European Conference on HIV/AIDS for the Muslim and South Asian Communities*, London, 1992.

NAZ Project, *Contexts – Report on Needs Assessment of Ethnic Minority Communities in Terms of HIV/AIDS*, London, 1992.

Ng'weshemi, Japheth, Boerma, Ties, Bennett, John and Schapink, Dick (eds), *HIV Prevention and AIDS Care in Africa: A District Level Approach*, The Netherlands, Royal Tropical Institute, 1997.

Panos Dossier No. 1, *AIDS and the Third World*, London, Panos Institute, 1986.

Panos Dossier No. 6, *The Hidden Cost of AIDS: The Challenge of HIV to Development*, London, Panos Institute, 1992.

Parker, Richard, 'Empowerment, community mobilization and social change in the face of HIV/AIDS', Vancouver, 9th International Conference on AIDS, July 1996 (unpublished).

Patton, Cindy, 'From nation to family: containing "African AIDS"', chap. 11 in Parker, Andrew, Russo, Mary, Sommer, Dorris and Yaeger, Patricia (eds), *Nationalisms and Sexualities*, London, Routledge, 1982.

Preble, E., Elias, C. and Winikoff, B., 'Maternal health in the age of AIDS: implications for health services in developing countries', in *AIDS Care*, 1994, 499–516.

Rader, Alison and Campbell, Ian, *Sustainability and Extension of Field Response to HIV/AIDS*, London, Salvation Army, 1994.

Scheper-Hughes, Nancy, 'AIDS and the social body', in *Social Science and Medicine*, 1994, 991–1003.

Sepulveda, James *et al.* (eds), *AIDS: Prevention through Education: A World View*, Oxford University Press, 1992.

Sieghard, Paul, *AIDS and Human Rights*, London, BMA Foundation for AIDS, 1989.

Sittitrai, Werasit and Williams, Glen, *Candles of Hope: The AIDS Programme of the Thai Red Cross Society*, London, ActionAid, 1994.

(2) AIDS, CHRISTIAN CHURCHES AND THEOLOGY

AIDS: Life and Love, Proceedings of the 10th Congress of Asian Federation of Catholic Medical Associations, Seoul, Korea, 1992.

Allen, Joseph, 'The Christian understanding of human relations: resource for the Churches' response to AIDS', in *The Ecumenical Review*, 1995, 353–63.

Bayley, Anne, *One New Humanity: The Challenge of AIDS*, London, SPCK, 1996.

Benn, Christoph and Boyd, Kenneth, 'Ethics, medical ethics and HIV/AIDS', in *The Ecumenical Review*, 1996, 222–32.

Bernardin, Cardinal Joseph, 'The Church's response to the AIDS crisis', in *Origins*, 13 November 1986, 383–5.

Catholic AIDS Link, *Positively Called – HIV, Priesthood and Religious Life (Pastoral Aids series, No. 2)*, London, Catholic AIDS Link, 1995.

Catholic AIDS Link, *Positive Reflections – Some Pastoral and Theological Resources (Pastoral Aids series, No. 3)*, London, Catholic AIDS Link, 1997.

Commission sociale de l'épiscopat (Albert Rouet, président), *SIDA, La société en question*, Paris, Bayard Editions/Centurion, 1996.

Dominian, Jack, 'AIDS and morality', in *The Tablet*, 10 January 1987, 33–4.

Fageol, Suzanne, 'The circle is cast: a feminist view of AIDS ministry', in *Feminist Theology*, 1993, 115–20.

Fitzpatrick, Bill *AIDS: Sharing the Pain*, London, Darton, Longman & Todd, 1988.

Fuller, Jon, *HIV/AIDS: An Overview*, Chicago, National Conference of Priests, 1995.

Fuller, Jon, 'AIDS prevention: a challenge to the Catholic moral tradition', in *America*, 28 December 1996, 13–20.

Fuller, Jon, O'Connor, Jay and Schexnayder, James, *Clergy and Religious and the AIDS Epidemic*, Chicago, National Federation of Priest Councils, October 1994, vol. V, no. 6.

Hannon, Patrick, 'AIDS: moral issues', in *Studies*, 1990, 103–15.

Hanvey, James, 'AIDS and ARC: a theological reflection on the Church's ministry', in *The Month*, December 1986, 326–31.

Jacobs, Michael, 'Considerations in the pastoral care of AIDS', in *Contact*, 1989, 2, 2–13.

John, T. Jacob, 'Sexuality, sin and disease: theological and ethical issues posed by AIDS to the churches: reflections by a physician', in *The Ecumenical Review*, 1995, 373–84.

Keenan, James F., 'Prophylactics, toleration and cooperation: contemporary problems and traditional principles', in *International Philosophical Quarterly*, 1989, 205–20.

Keenan, James F., 'HIV testing of seminary and religious-order candidates', in *Review for Religious*, May–June 1996, 297–314.

Kelly, David, 'Condoms and AIDS in Catholic hospitals', in his *Critical Care Ethics: Treatment Decisions in American Hospitals*, Kansas City, Sheed & Ward, 1991, 204–8.

Kelly, Kevin, *Diary of Visit to Uganda*, June–July 1994 (unpublished).

Kelly, Kevin, *Diary of Visit to Bangkok and Manila*, Jan–Feb, 1995 (unpublished).

Kirkpatrick, Bill (ed.), *Cry Love, Cry Hope: Responding to AIDS*, London, Darton, Longman & Todd, 1994.

Kowalewski, Mark, *All Things to All People: The Catholic Church Confronts the AIDS Crisis*, New York, New York State University Press, 1994.

Lindsey, William D., 'The AIDS crisis and the Church: a time to heal,' in *Theology and Sexuality*, no. 2, March 1995, 11–37.

Logie, Dorothy, 'Your law or my life', in *The Tablet*, 8 March 1997, 314.

McCormick, Richard A. 'AIDS: the shape of the ethical challenge', in *America*, 13 February 1988, 147–54.

McDonagh, Enda, 'Theology in a time of AIDS', in *Irish Theological Quarterly*, 1994, 81–99 and reprinted in his *Faith in Fragments*, Maynooth Bicentenary Series, Dublin, Columba Press, 1996.

MacLaren, Duncan (ed.), *The Church Responds to HIV/AIDS*, London, CAFOD/Caritas Internationalis, 1996.

McNeill, John, 'The gay response to AIDS: becoming a resurrection people', in *The Way*, 1987, 332–41.

Morton, Gillian, 'AIDS and the Scottish Churches', in *Contact*, 1989, 2, 9–13.

New Blackfriars, Special Issue: *Christians and AIDS: An Anglo-French Assessment*, August 1990.

Nicolson, Ronald, *AIDS: A Christian Response*, Pietermaritzburg, South Africa, Cluster Publications, 1995.

Nicolson, Ronald, *God in AIDS?*, London, SCM, 1996.

Northcott, Michael S., *AIDS, Sex and the Scottish Churches*, Edinburgh, Centre for Theology and Public Issues, 1993.

O'Donohue, Maura and Vitillo, Robert, 'HIV tests for candidates?', in *Religious Life Review*, 1992, 160–2.

Overberg, Kenneth R., *AIDS: Ethics and Religion: Embracing a World of Suffering*, New York, Orbis, 1994.

Paterson, Gillian, *Love in a Time of AIDS: Women, Health and the Challenge of HIV*, Geneva, WCC Publications and New York, Orbis, 1996.

Pattison, Stephen, 'The judgement of AIDS', in *Contact*, 1989, 3, 26–32.

Regan, Dennis M., *Special Moral Issues*, in Robert J. Vitillo (ed.), *The Pandemic of Aids*, Caritas Internationalis/CAFOD, 1988, 58–67.

Reiter, Johannes, 'AIDS: the virus and moral', in *Theology Digest*, 1988, 3–8.

Rotter, Hans, 'AIDS: some theological and pastoral considerations', in *Theology Digest*, Fall 1992, 1235–9.

Russell, Letty M. (ed.), *The Church with AIDS*, Louisville, KY, Westminster Press, 1990.

Shelp, Earl E. and Sutherland, Ronald H., *AIDS and the Church: The Second Decade*, Louisville, KY, Westminster/John Knox Press, 1992.

Smith, Richard L., *AIDS, Gays and the American Catholic Church*, Cleveland, OH, The Pilgrim Press, 1994.

Thampu, Valson, *AIDS: Heresy and Prophecy: What the Virus Says*, New Delhi, Theological Research and Communication Institute, 1993.

US Bishops' Conference 'The many faces of AIDS: a gospel response', in *Origins*, 24 December 1987, 481–9; 'Called to compassion and responsibility: a response to the HIV/AIDS crisis', in *Origins*, 30 November 1989, 421–36.

Winfield, Flora, '"For nothing can separate us from the love of Christ" – Who does belong to the body of Christ?', in *The Ecumenical Review*, 1995, 364–72.

World Council of Churches Study Document, *Facing AIDS: The Challenge, the Churches' Response*, Geneva, WCC Publications, 1997.

Woodward, James (ed.), *Embracing the Chaos: Theological Responses to AIDS*, London, SPCK, 1991.

Woodward, James, 'AIDS: the crisis and the opportunities', in *Contact*, 1990, 1, 15–19.

(3) WOMEN AND AIDS

Berer, Marge with Ray, Sunanda (eds), *Women and HIV/AIDS: an International Resource Book*, London, Pandora, 1993.

Fageol, Suzanne, 'The circle is cast: a feminist view of AIDS ministry', in *Feminist Theology*, 1993, 115–20.

Farmer, Paul, Connors, Margaret and Simmons, Janie (eds), *Women, Poverty and AIDS: Sex, Drugs and Structural Violence*, Monroe, ME, Common Courage Press, 1996.

Gorna, Robin, *Vamps, Virgins and Victims: How Can Women Fight AIDS?*, London, Cassell, 1996.

Kaleeba, Noerine, *We Miss You All*, Harare, Zimbabwe, Women & AIDS Support Network, 1991.

Logie, Dorothy, 'Women & AIDS in Uganda', in *MedicalWOMAN*, Summer 1995, 8–9.

Mertz, David *et al.*, 'Women and AIDS: the ethics of exaggerated harm', in *Bioethics*, 1996, 93–113.

Panos Dossier No. 4, *Triple Jeopardy: Women and AIDS*, London, Panos Institute, 1990.

Paterson, Gillian, *Love in a Time of AIDS: Women, Health and the Challenge of HIV*, Geneva, WCC Publications and New York, Orbis, 1996.

Patton, Cindy, *Last Served? Gendering the HIV Pandemic*, London, Taylor & Francis, 1994.

Sherr, Lorraine, Hankins, Catherine and Bennett, Lydia, *AIDS as a Gender Issue: Psychosocial Perspectives*, London, Taylor & Francis, 1996.

Shroff, F. M. 'The social construction of AIDS, heterosexism, racism and misogyny: and the challenges facing women of colour', in *RFR/DRF*, vol. 20, no. 3/4 (1991),115–23.

UN Development Programme, *Changing the Focus*, New York, United Nations, no date.

World Health Organization and the UN Development Programme in consultation with the UN Division for the Advancement of Women, *Women and AIDS*, New York, United Nations, 1994.

(4) WOMEN VIS–À–VIS THE CHURCHES, THEOLOGY AND SOCIETY

Books

Becher, Jeanne (ed.), *Women, Religion and Sexuality: Studies on the Impact of Religious Teachings on Women*, Geneva, WCC Publications, 1990.

Borrowdale, Anne, *Distorted Images: Christian Attitudes to Women, Men and Sex*, London, SPCK, 1991.

Brown, Joanne Carlson, and Bohn, Carole R. (eds), *Christianity, Patriarchy and Abuse: A Feminist Critique*, Cleveland, OH, The Pilgrim Press, 1989.

Brown, Peter, *The Body and Society: Men, Women and Sexual Renunciation in Early Christianity*, London, Faber & Faber, 1988.

Cahill, Lisa Sowle, *Women and Sexuality*, New York, Paulist Press, 1992.

Cahill, Lisa Sowle, *Sex, Gender and Christian Ethics*, Cambridge University Press, 1996.

Carr, Anne E., *Liberating Conscience: Feminist Explorations in Catholic Moral Theology*, London, SCM, 1996.

Carr, Anne E., *Transforming Grace: Christian Tradition and Women's Experience*, London, HarperCollins, 1988.

Chittister, Joan, *Beyond Beijing: The Next Step for Women*, Kansas City, Sheed & Ward, 1996.

Elwes, Teresa (ed.), *Women's Voices: Essays in Contemporary Feminist Theology*, London, Marshall Pickering, 1992.

Fiorenza, Elisabeth Schüssler, and Copeland, Mary Shawn (eds), *Violence against Women: Concilium 1994/1*, London, SCM, 1994.

Gnanadason, Aruna, *No Longer a Secret: The Church and Violence against Women*, Geneva, WCC Publications, 1993.

Graham, Elaine, *Making the Difference: Gender, Personhood and Theology*, London, Mowbray, 1995.

Grey, Mary, *Redeeming the Dream: Feminism, Redemption and Christian Tradition*, London, SPCK, 1989.

Grey, Mary, *The Wisdom of Fools? Seeking Revelation for Today*, London, SPCK, 1993.

Gryson R., *The Ministry of Women in the Early Church*, Collegeville, MN, The Liturgical Press, 1976.

Halkes, Catharina J. M., *New Creation: Christian Feminism and the Renewal of the Earth*, London, SPCK, 1991.

Hunt, Mary E., *Fierce Tenderness: A Feminist Theology of Friendship*, New York, Crossroad, 1992.

Johnson, Elizabeth A., *She Who Is: The Mystery of God in Feminist Theological Discourse*, New York, Crossroad, 1995.

Mananzan, Mary John, *The Woman Question in the Philippines*, Manila, St Paul, 1991.

Moltmann-Wendel, Elisabeth, *I Am My Body: New Ways of Embodiment*, London, SCM, 1994.

Oduyoye, Mercy Amba, *Daughters of Anowa: African Women and Patriarchy*, New York, Orbis, 1995.

Parsons, Susan Frank, *Feminism and Christian Ethics*, Cambridge University Press, 1996.

Patrick, Anne E., *Liberating Conscience: Feminist Explorations in Catholic Moral Theology*, London, SCM, 1996.

Plaskow, Judith and Christ, Carol P. (eds), *Weaving the Visions: New Patterns in Feminist Spirituality*, San Francisco, Harper & Row, 1989.

Power, Kim, *Veiled Desire: Augustine's Writing on Women*, London, Darton, Longman & Todd, 1995.

Radcliffe Richards, Janet, *The Sceptical Feminist: A Philosophical Enquiry*, London, Penguin, new edn, 1994.

Ruether, Rosemary Radford, *Sexism and God-Talk: Towards a Feminist Theology*, London, SCM, 1983.

Thistlethwaite, Susan, *Sex, Race, and God: Christian Feminism in Black and White*, London, Geoffrey Chapman, 1990.

Thurston, Anne, *Because of Her Testimony: The Word in Female Experience*, Dublin, Gill & Macmillan, 1995.

Webster, Alison, *Found Wanting: Women, Christianity and Sexuality*, London, Cassell, 1995.

Articles in periodicals, etc.

Al-Touqatchi, Yasmin, 'The diary of an unconcerned woman', in *Feminist Theology*, 1993, 26–31.

Andolsen, Barbara Hilkert, 'Gender and sex roles in recent religious ethics literature', in *Religious Studies Review*, 1985, 217–23.

Beya, Bernadette Mbua, 'Ways to liberate the women of Africa', in *The Tablet*, 14 May 1994, 591–2.

Cahill, Lisa Sowle, 'Feminist ethics', in *Theological Studies*, 1990, 49–64.

Cahill, Lisa Sowle, 'Feminist ethics and the challenge of cultures', 1993 Presidential Address, in *Proceedings of the Catholic Theological Society of America*, 1993, 65–83.

Conn, Joann Wolsk, 'New vitality: the challenge from feminist theology', in *America*, 5 October 1991, 217–19.

Donovan, Mary Ann, 'Women's issues: an agenda for the Church?', in *Horizons*, 1987, 283–95.

Gillis, Chester, 'Feminist theology, Roman Catholicism, and alienation', in *Horizons*, 1993, 280–300.

Glendon, Professor Mary Ann (Head of Holy See's Delegation at Beijing Conference), *Opening Address at Conference*, text in *Briefing*, 19 October 1995, 16–19.

Graham, Elaine, 'From space to woman-space', in *Feminist Theology*, 1995, 10–34.

Grey, Mary, 'Has feminist theology a vision for the Christian Church?', in *Louvain Studies*, 1991, 17–40.

Gudorf, Christine, 'Women's choice for motherhood: beginning a cross-cultural approach in motherhood', in *Concilium*, no. 206, 55–63.

John Paul II, *Letter to Women*, text in *The Tablet*, 15 July 1985, 917–21; Message of 26 May 1995 to the UN 1995 Conference on Women at Beijing presented to its Secretary General, Mrs Gertrude Mongella (text in *Briefing*, 17 August 1995, 16–18); Allocution in Rome, in *L'Osservatore Romano*, English edition, 6 September 1995.

Kahoe, Richard D., 'Social science of gender differences: ideological battleground', in *Religious Studies Review*, 1985, 223–8.

Leonard, Ellen, 'Experience as a source for theology', in 'The sources of theology' in *Proceedings of the Catholic Theological Society in America*, 1988, 44–61.

Meyer-Wilmes, Hedwig, 'Woman's nature and feminine identity. Theological legitimations and feminist questions', in *Concilium*, no. 194, 93–101.

Miller, Annabel, 'Women in the Vatican', in *The Tablet*, 29 March / 2 April 1997, 428–30.

Pellauer, Mary D., 'The moral significance of female orgasm: towards sexual ethics that celebrates women's sexuality', in Nelson, James B. and Longfellow, Sandra P. (eds), *Sexuality and the Sacred: Sources for Theological Reflection*, London, Mowbray, 1994, 149–68.

Pfäfflin, Ursula, 'Mothers in a patriarchal world: experience and feminist theory', in *Concilium*, no. 206, 15–22.

Pollitt, Katha, 'Are women morally superior to men?', in *The Nation*, 28 December 1992, 799–807.

Ruether, Rosemary Radford, 'The development of my theology', in *Religious Studies Review*, 1989, 1–11.

Saiving, Valerie, 'The human situation: a feminine view', in Christ, C. and Plaskow, J. (eds), *Womanspirit Rising: A Feminist Reader in Religion*, San Francisco, Harper & Row, 1979, 25–42.

Secker, Susan L., 'Human experience and women's experience: resources for Christian ethics', in *Annual of Society of Christian Ethics*, 1991, 133–50.

Society of Jesus, 'Jesuits and the situation of women in Church and civil society', in *Documents of the 34th General Congregation of the Society of Jesus*, Saint Louis, Institute of Jesuit Sources, 1995, 174–6.

Zappone, Katherine, '"Woman's special nature": a different horizon for theological anthropology', in *Concilium*, 1991/1, 87–97.

(5) SEXUAL ETHICS

Official or semi-official church reports

British Council of Churches (BCC) Working Party Report, *Sex and Morality*, 1966. (See also under Moss, Rachel.)

CDF (Congregation for the Doctrine of the Faith), *Declaration on Certain Questions Concerning Sexual Ethics* (1975).

Church of England Reports: *The Family in Contemporary Society* (1958); *Putting Asunder: A Divorce Law for a Contemporary Society* (1966); *Marriage, Divorce and the Church* (1972); *Marriage and the Church's Task* (1978); *Homosexual Relationships* (1979); *An Honourable Estate* (1988); *Issues in Human Sexuality* (1991); *Something to Celebrate: Valuing Families in Church and Society* (1995).

Church of Scotland, 1994 General Assembly, Report of the Panel on Doctrine Working Party, 'On the theology of marriage'; and Report from the Board of Social Responsibility, 'Human sexuality' (texts in *The Church of Scotland: Reports to the General Assembly*, 1994, 257–85 and 500–16).

Durber, Susan (ed.), *As Man and Woman Made: Theological Reflections on Marriage* (Report from United Reformed Church's Doctrine and Worship Committee), London, United Reformed Church, 1994.

Evangelical Lutheran Church in America, *The Church and Human Sexuality: A Lutheran Perspective: First Draft of a Social Statement*, Minneapolis, MN, ECLA Distribution Service, 1993.

Methodist Church, 1939 Conference statement, *The Christian View of Marriage and the Family*; Division of Social Responsibility Reports to Conference, *A Christian Understanding of Human Sexuality* (1980 and 1982 Reports); Division of Social Responsibility, *Report of Commission on Human Sexuality* (1990).

Moss, Rachel (ed.) (British Council of Churches Working Party), *God's Yes to Sexuality*, London, Collins, 1981.

Pontifical Council for the Family, 'Vademecum for confessors on some themes of conjugal morality' (12 February 1997), in *Briefing*, 20 March 1997, 30–9.

Presbyterian Church (USA), *Decisions of the 203rd General Assembly on Human Sexuality: Response to the Report of a Special Committee on Human Sexuality, 'Keeping Body and Soul Together: Sexuality, Spirituality and Social Justice'*; and *Report of the Special Committee on Human Sexuality*, Louisville, KY, Office of the General Assembly, Presbyterian Church (USA), 1991.

Smith, Robin, *Living in Covenant with God and One Another: A Guide to the Study of Sexuality and Human Relations Using Statements from WCC Member Churches*, Geneva, WCC Publications, 1990.

Society of Friends, *Towards a Quaker View of Sex: An Essay by a Group of Friends*, London, Friends Home Service Committee, 1963.

Uniting Church in Australia, Assembly Task Group on Sexuality, *Uniting Sexuality and Faith*, Collingwood, Australia, The Joint Board of Christian Education, 1997.

Books

Blenkinsopp, Joseph, *Sexuality and the Christian Tradition*, London, Sheed & Ward, 1970.

Brett, Paul, *Rethinking Christian Attitudes to Sex*, Colchester, Centre for the Study of Theology in the University of Essex (Essex Papers in Theology and Society, no. 4), 1991.

Brown, Peter, *The Body and Society: Men, Women and Sexual Renunciation in Early Christianity*, London, Faber & Faber, 1988.

Cahill, Lisa Sowle, *Between the Sexes*, Philadelphia, Fortress Press, 1985.

Cahill, Lisa Sowle, *Women and Sexuality*, New York, Paulist Press, 1992.

Cahill, Lisa Sowle, *Sex, Gender and Christian Ethics*, Cambridge University Press, 1996.

Carey, John J. (ed.), *The Sexuality Debate in North American Churches, 1988–1995: Controversies, Unresolved Issues, Future Prospects*, Lampeter, Dyfed, Edwin Mellen Press, 1995.

Coleman, Gerald D., *Human Sexuality: An All-Embracing Gift*, New York, Alba House, 1992.

Countryman, L. William, *Dirt, Greed and Sex: Sexual Ethics in the New Testament and Their Implications for Today*, London, SCM, 1989.

Cross Currents, vol. 14, n. 2 (Spring 1964) – special edition: *Sexuality in the Modern World*.

Curran, Charles, *Issues in Sexual and Medical Ethics*, Indiana, University of Notre Dame Press, 1978.

Curran, Charles E. and McCormick, Richard A. (eds), *Dialogue about Catholic Sexual Teaching (Readings in Moral Theology No. 8)*, New York, Paulist Press, 1993.

Davies, Jon and Loughlin, Gerard (eds), *Sex These Days: Essays on Theology, Sexuality and Society*, Sheffield, Sheffield Academic Press, 1997.

De Locht, Pierre, *Morale sexuelle et magistère*, Paris, Éditions du Cerf, 1992.

Dominian, Jack, *Proposals for a New Sexual Ethic*, London, Darton, Longman & Todd, 1977.

Dominian, Jack, *Sexual Integrity: The Answer to AIDS*, London, Darton, Longman & Todd, 1987.

Dominian, Jack and Montefiore, Hugh, *God, Sex and Love*, London, SCM, 1989.

Farley, Margaret A., *Personal Commitments: Beginning, Keeping, Changing*, San Francisco, Harper & Row, 1990.

Fuchs, Eric, *Sexual Desire and Love: Origins and History of the Christian Ethic of Sexuality and Marriage*, Cambridge, James Clarke, 1983.

Galloway, Kathy (ed.), *Dreaming of Eden: Reflections on Christianity and Sexuality*, Glasgow, Wild Goose Publications, 1997.

Genovesi, Vincent J., *In Pursuit of Love: Catholic Morality and Human Sexuality*, Dublin, Gill & Macmillan, 1987.

Gosling, J., *Marriage and the Love of God*, London, Geoffrey Chapman, 1965.

Gudorf, Christine, *Reconstructing Christian Sexual Ethics: Body, Sex and Pleasure as Grace and Gift*, Cleveland, OH, The Pilgrim Press, 1994.

Guindon, André, *The Sexual Language*, Ottawa, University of Ottawa Press, 1977.

Guindon, André, *The Sexual Creators: An Ethical Proposal for Concerned Christians*, New York, University Press of America, 1986.

Hanigan, James P., *What Are They Saying about Sexual Morality?*, New York, Paulist Press, 1982.

Harvey, Anthony, *Promise or Pretence? A Christian Guide to Sexual Morals*, London, SCM, 1994.

Heyward, Carter, *Our Passion for Justice: Images of Power, Sexuality and Liberation*, Cleveland, OH, The Pilgrim Press, 1984.

Heyward, Carter, *Touching Our Strength: The Erotic as Power and the Love of God*, San Francisco, Harper & Row, 1989.

Heyward, Carter, *Staying Power: Reflections on Gender, Justice and Compassion*, Cleveland, OH, The Pilgrim Press, 1995.

Keane, Philip S., *Sexual Morality: A Catholic Perspective*, Dublin, Gill & Macmillan, 1977.

Kosnik, A. (ed.), *Human Sexuality: New Directions in Catholic Thought*, London, Search Press, 1977.

Markman, Howard, Stanley, Scott and Blumberg, Susan L., *Fighting for Your Marriage: Positive Steps for Preventing Divorce and Preserving a Lasting Love*, San Francisco, Jossey-Bass, 1994.

Moore, Gareth, *The Body in Context: Sex and Catholicism*, London, SCM, 1992.

Nelson, James B., *Embodiment: An Approach to Sexuality and Christian Theology*, London, SPCK, 1978.

Nelson, James B., *Between Two Gardens: Reflections on Sexuality and Religious Experience*, New York, Pilgrim Press, 1983.

Nelson, James B. (ed.), *Sexual Ethics and the Church*, Chicago, IL, The Christian Century Foundation, 1989.

Nelson, James B., *The Intimate Connection: Male Sexuality, Masculine Spirituality*, London, SPCK, 1992.

Nelson, James B. and Longfellow, Sandra P. (eds), *Sexuality and the Sacred: Sources for Theological Reflection*, London, Mowbray, 1994.

Oppenheimer, Helen, *Marriage*, London, Mowbray, 1990.

Reidy, Maurice, *Freedom to be Friends: Morals and Sexual Affection*, London, Collins, 1990.

Roberts, William P. (ed.), *Commitment to Partnership: Explorations of the Theology of Marriage*, New York, Paulist Press, 1987.

Schillebeeckx, Edward, *Marriage: Secular Reality and Saving Mystery*, vol. 1, London, Sheed & Ward, 1965.

Scruton, Roger, *Sexual Desire: A Philosophical Investigation*, London, Weidenfeld & Nicolson, 1986.

Sexuality and Spirituality, special issue of *The Way*, July 1988.

Spong, John Shelby, *Living in Sin: A Bishop Rethinks Human Sexuality*, San Francisco, Harper & Row, 1988.

Storkey, Elaine, *The Search for Intimacy*, London, Hodder & Stoughton, 1995.

Studies in Christian Ethics, vol. 4, no. 2 – special issue on Sexual Ethics.

Stuart, Elizabeth, and Thatcher, Adrian, *People of Passion: What the Churches Teach about Sex*, London, Mowbray, 1997.

Thatcher, Adrian, *Liberating Sex: A Christian Sexual Theology*, London, SPCK, 1993.

Thatcher, Adrian, and Stuart, Elizabeth, *Christian Perspectives on Sexuality and Gender*, Leominster, Gracewing, 1996.

Timmerman, Joan H., *Sexuality and Spiritual Growth*, New York, Crossroad, 1992.

Trible, Phyllis, *God and the Rhetoric of Sexuality*, London, SCM, 1992.

Weeks, Jeffrey, *Sexuality and Its Discontents: Means, Myths and Modern Sexualities*, London, Routledge & Kegan Paul, 1985.

Whitehead, E. and Whitehead, J. D., *A Sense of Sexuality: Christian Love and Intimacy*, New York, Doubleday, 1989.

Articles in periodicals, etc.

Anscombe, G. E. M., 'You can have sex without children: Christianity and the new offer', in her *Collected Philosophical Papers III: Ethics, Religion and Politics*, Oxford, Blackwell, 1981, 84–96.

Au, Wilkie, 'Sexuality in the service of life and love', in his book, *By Way of the Heart: Towards a Holistic Christian Spirituality*, London, Geoffrey Chapman, 1990, chap. 6.

Banner, Michael, 'Five Churches in search of sexual ethics: a short commentary on a statement from the House of Bishops and some other recent reports', in *Theology*, 1993, 276–89.

Barton, Stephen C., 'Is the Bible good news for human sexuality? Reflections on method in biblical interpretation', in *Theology and Sexuality*, September 1994, 42–54.

Cahill, Lisa Sowle, 'Sexual ethics', in Macquarrie, John and Childress,

James (eds), *A New Dictionary of Christian Ethics*, London, SCM, 1986, 579–83.

Cahill, Lisa Sowle, 'On the connection of sex to reproduction', in Shelp, Earl (ed.), *Sexuality and Medicine, vol II, Ethical Viewpoints in Transition*, Dordrecht, Kluwer Academic Publishers, 1987, 39–50.

Cahill, Lisa Sowle, 'Sexuality, marriage and parenthood: the Catholic tradition', in Shannon, Thomas and Cahill, Lisa Sowle, *Religion and Artifical Reproduction*, New York, Crossroad, 1988, chap. 2.

Cahill, Lisa Sowle, 'Human sexuality', in Curran, Charles (ed.), *Moral Theology: Challenges for the Future*, New York, Paulist Press, 1990, chap. 10.

Cahill, Lisa Sowle, *Sex and Gender: Catholic Teaching and the Signs of Our Times*, unpublished lecture, Dublin, 1994.

Callaghan, Brendan, 'Idolatry and intimacy: thoughts towards a synthesis on sexuality', in *Theology and Sexuality*, no. 1, 1994, 96–105.

Clarke, Katherine M., 'Dimensions of human relationship', in *Human Development*, Fall 1996, 5–11.

Connors, Russell B. Jnr., 'Towards consistent Catholic ethics: a different dialogue partner for sexual morality', in *Irish Theological Quarterly*, 1995, 219–34.

Deidun, Thomas, 'Beyond dualisms', in *The Way*, July 1988, 195–205 (on Paul).

Dowell, Susan, 'Challenging monogamy', in *Theology and Sexuality*, March 1995, 84–103.

Ellison, Marvin M., 'Common decency: a new Christian sexual ethics', in *Common Sense*, March 1991, 8–12.

Farley, Margaret A., 'Sexual ethics', in Reich, Warren T. (ed.), *Encyclopedia of Bioethics*, vol. IV, New York, Macmillan, The Free Press, 1978, 1575–87.

Fox, Robin, 'The conditions of sexual evolution', in Aries, Philippe and Bejin, Andre (eds), *Western Sexuality: Practice and Precept in Past and Present Times*, Oxford, Blackwell, 1985, chap. 1.

Francoeur, Robert T., 'New dimensions in human sexuality', in Iles, Robert H. (ed.), *The Gospel Imperative in the Midst of AIDS*, Wilton, CT, Morehouse, 1989, 79–105.

Gleeson, G. P., 'Procreation and sexual desire', in *Irish Theological Quarterly*, 1988, 190–210.

Grisewood, Harman, 'On human sexuality', in *The Tablet*, 1 March 1997, 286–7.

Gudorf, Christine E. and Blaney, Robert W., 'Recent works on Christian sexual ethics', in *Religious Studies Review*, April 1988, 125–31.

Guindon, André, 'L'Être-femme: deux lectures', in *Église et Théologie*, 1978, 103–68.

Guindon, André, 'Pour une fécondité sexuelle humaine', in *Science et Esprit*, 1981, 29–54.

Guindon, André, 'Le Témoignage sexuel des personnes ages', in *Église et Théologie*, 1985, 107–33.

Guindon, André, 'Sexual acts or sexual lifestyles? A methodological problem in sexual ethics', in *Église et théologie*, 1987, 315–40.

Guindon, André, 'Mentioning the unmentionables', in *Compass*, July 1989, 6–10.

Guindon, André, 'Theologian offers Vatican-requested explanations', in *Origins*, 25 February 1993, 630–6.

Guindon, André, 'Le Sens chrétien de la sexualité', in *Communauté Chrétienne*, n. 101, 444–52.

Harrison, Beverly Wildung, 'Human sexuality and mutuality', in Weidman, Judith L. (ed.), *Christian Feminism: Visions of a New Humanity*, San Francisco, Harper & Row, 1984, 141–57.

Harvey, A. E., 'Marriage, sex and Bible I & II', in *Theology*, 1993, 364–72 & 461–8.

Heyward, Carter, 'Sexuality, Love and Justice', in Plaskow, Judith and Christ, Carol, *Weaving the Visions: New Patterns in Feminist Spirituality*, San Francisco, Harper & Row, 1989, 293–301.

Hoose, Bernard, 'Theological trends – sexual ethics: some recent developments', in *The Way*, January 1993, 54–62.

Jones, Gareth, 'God's passionate embrace: notes for a Christian understanding of sexuality', in *Studies in Christian Ethics*, vol. 5, no. 2, 32–45.

Kolakowski, Victoria S., 'Toward a Christian ethical response to transsexual persons', in *Theology and Sexuality*, March 1997, 10–31.

Lacroix, Xavier, 'Une parole sur la sexualité au temps du sida', in *Études*, 1993, 483–93.

Lonergan, Bernard, 'Finality, Love, Marriage', in *Theological Studies*, 1943, 477–510.

Lorde, Audre, 'Uses of the erotic: the erotic as power', in her *Sister Outsider: Essays and Speeches*, Trumansburg, NY, Crossing Press, 1984, 52–9.

Miller, Annabel, 'Casualties of the sexual revolution', in *The Tablet*, 18 May 1996.

Moore, Gareth, 'Sex, sexuality and relationships', in Hoose, Bernard, *Christian Ethics: An Introduction*, London, Cassell, 1998, 223–47.

Nelson, James B., ' On doing body theology', in *Theology and Sexuality*, March 1995, 38–60.

O'Connell, Timothy E., 'Sexuality and the procreative norm', in Greenspahn, F. (ed.), *Contemporary Ethical Issues in Jewish and Christian Traditions*, Hoboken, New Jersey, Ktav Publishing House, 1985, 81–109.

Parmisano, Fabiano, 'Love and marriage in the Middle Ages', in *New Blackfriars*, 1969, 599–608 & 649–60.

Price, Richard, 'The distinctiveness of early Christian sexual ethics', in *Heythrop Journal*, 1990, 257–76.

Radcliffe, Timothy, '"Glorify God in your bodies": I Cor 6.12–20 as a sexual ethic', in *New Blackfriars*, 1986, 306–14.

Selling, Joseph, 'Evolution and continuity in conjugal morality', in Selling, J. A. (ed.), *Personalist Ethics: Essays in Honour of Professor Louis Janssens*, Leuven, Leuven University Press, 1988, 243–64.

Selling, Joseph, 'On sex and sexuality: the challenge of André Guindon', in *Doctrine and Life*, January 1993, 31–41.

Shanks, Norman, 'Imprisoned by fear? The Church of Scotland's debate about human sexuality', in *Theology and Sexuality*, September 1995, 77–97.

Thatcher, Adrian, 'Singles and/or families . . . ', in *Theology and Sexuality*, March 1996, 11–27.

Thompsett, Fredrica Harris, 'Power in flesh: incarnational perspectives on intimacy', in her *Courageous Incarnation: in Intimacy, Work, Childhood and Aging*, Cambridge, Boston, Cowley Publications, 1993, 126–58.

Williams, Rowan, *The Body's Grace* (10th Michael Harding Memorial Lecture), London, Lesbian and Gay Christian Movement, 1989.

(6) HOMOSEXUALITY

Official or semi-official Church reports

Catholic Bishops of Washington State, *The Prejudice against Homosexuals and the Ministry of the Church* (1983).

Catholic Social Welfare Commission of the Bishops' Conference of England and Wales, *An Introduction to the Pastoral Care of Homosexual People* (1979).

Church of England, Board for Social Responsibility, *Homosexuality. A Contribution to Discussion* (1979).

Congregation for the Doctrine of the Faith, *Letter to the Bishops of the Catholic Church on the Pastoral Care of Homosexual Persons* (1986).

Congregation for the Doctrine of the Faith, *Letter to U.S. Bishops: Some Considerations Concerning the Response to Legislative Proposals on the Non-discrimination of Homosexual Persons* (25 June 1992).

Hume, Cardinal Basil, *A Note on the Teaching of the Catholic Church Concerning Homosexual People*, February 1995 (revised April 1997).

United Reformed Church Working Party, *Homosexuality: A Christian View* (1991).

US National Conference of Catholic Bishops Committee, 'Pastoral message to parents of homosexual children and suggestions for pastoral ministers', in *Origins*, 9 October 1997, 285–91.

Cf. also Official and Semi-Official Church Reports listed in Bibliography, section 5 above.

Books

Bailey, Sherwin, *Homosexuality and the Western Christian Tradition*, London, Longmans, 1955.

Batchelor, Edward (ed.), *Homosexuality and Ethics*, New York, Pilgrim Press, 1980.

Bathurst Gilson, Anne, *Eros Breaking Free: Interpreting Sexual Theo-Ethics*, Cleveland, OH, The Pilgrim Press, 1995.

Boswell, John, *Christianity, Social Tolerance and Homosexuality: Gay People in Western Europe*, Chicago, IL, University of Chicago Press, 1980.

Bouldrey, Brian (ed.), *Wrestling with the Angel: Faith and Religion in the Lives of Gay Men*, New York, Riverhead Books, 1995.

Bradshaw, Timothy (ed.), *The Way Forward? Christian Voices on Homosexuality and the Church*, London, Hodder & Stoughton, 1997.

Brash, Alan, *Facing Our Differences: The Churches and Their Gay and Lesbian Members*, Geneva, WCC Publications, 1995.

Burr, Chandler, *A Separate Creation: How Biology Makes Us Gay*, London, Bantam Press, 1996.

Coleman, Peter, *Christian Attitudes to Homosexuality*, London, SPCK, 1980.

Coleman, Peter, *Gay Christians: a Moral Dilemma*, London, SCM, 1989.

Comstock, Gary, *Gay Theology without Apology*, Cleveland, OH, The Pilgrim Press, 1993.

Davies, P. M., Hickson, F. C. I., Weatherburn, P. and Hunt, A. J., *Sex, Gay Men and AIDS* (Social Aspects of AIDS series), London, The Falmer Press, 1993.

Goss, Robert, *Jesus Acted Up: A Gay and Lesbian Manifesto*, San Francisco, Harper & Row, 1993.

Gramick, Jeannine and Furey, Pat (eds), *The Vatican and Homosexuality: Reactions to the 'Letter to the Bishops of the Catholic Church on the Pastoral Care of Homosexual Persons'*, New York, Crossroad, 1988.

Gramick, Jeannine (ed.), *Homosexuality in the Priesthood and the Religious Life*, New York, Crossroad, 1989.

Gramick, Jeannine and Nugent, Robert (eds), *Voices of Hope: A Collection of Positive Catholic Writings on Gay and Lesbian Issues*, New York, Center for Homophobia Education, 1995.

Helminiak, Daniel A., *What the Bible Really Says about Homosexuality*, San Francisco, Alamo Square Press, 1994.

Jung, Patricia and Smith, Ralph, *Heterosexism: An Ethical Challenge*, New York, State University of New York Press, 1993.

LeVay, Simon, *Queer Science: The Use and Abuse of Research into Homosexuality*, Cambridge, MA, The MIT Press, 1996.

McNeill, John, *The Church and the Homosexual*, Boston, Beacon Press, 4th edn, 1993.

McNeill, John, *Freedom Glorious Freedom: The Spiritual Journey to the Fullness of Life for Gays, Lesbians and Everybody Else*, Boston, Beacon Press, 1995.

Moberly, Elizabeth, *Homosexuality: A New Christian Ethic*, Cambridge, James Clarke, 1983.

Nugent, Robert (ed.), *A Challenge to Love: Gay and Lesbian Catholics in the Church*, New York, Crossroad, 1989.

Nugent, Robert and Gramick, Jeannine, *Building Bridges: Gay and Lesbian Reality and the Catholic Church*, Mystic, CT, Twenty-Third Publications, 1992.

Peddicord, Richard, *Gay and Lesbian Rights: A Question: Sexual Ethics or Sexual Justice?*, Kansas, Sheed & Ward, 1996.

Pharr, Suzanne, *Homophobia: A Weapon of Sexism*, Little Rock, AR, Chardon Press, 1988.

Pronk, Pim, *Against Nature? Types of Moral Argumentation Regarding Homosexuality*, Grand Rapids, MI, Eerdmans, 1993.

Rotello, Gabriel, *Sexual Ecology: AIDS and the Destiny of Gay Men*, New York: Dutton-Penguin, 1997.

Ruse, Michael, *Homosexuality: A Philosophical Enquiry*, Oxford, Basil Blackwell, 1988.

Scanzoni, Letha and Mollenkott, Virginia Ramey, *Is the Homosexual My Neighbour? Another Christian View*, London, SCM, 1978.

Scroggs, R., *The New Testament and Homosexuality: Contextual Background for Contemporary Debate*, Philadelphia, Fortress Press, 1985.

Shinnick, Maurice, *This Remarkable Gift*, St Leonard's, NSW, Allen & Unwin, 1997.

Stuart, Elizabeth, *Just Good Friends: Towards a Lesbian and Gay Theology of Relationships*, London, Mowbray, 1995.

Sullivan, Andrew, *Virtually Normal: An Argument about Homosexuality*, London, Picador, 1995.

Vasey, Michael, *Strangers and Friends: A New Exploration of Homosexuality and the Bible*, London, Hodder & Stoughton, 1995.

Articles in periodicals, etc.

Acceptance, Australia, *Letter on Pastoral Care of Gay Persons*, 1990.

Brubaker, Pamela K., 'A terror of touch: homosexuality debates in the Churches', in *Theology and Sexuality*, March 1997, 56–70.

Cahill, Lisa Sowle, 'Moral methodology: a case study', in Hamel, Ronald P. and Himes, Kenneth R. (eds), *Introduction to Christian Ethics: A Reader*, New York, Paulist Press, 1989, chap. 43.

Coleman, John, 'The homosexual revolution and hermeneutics', in *Concilium*, no. 173, 55–64.

Curran, Charles, 'Dialogue with the homophile movement: the morality of homosexuality', in his *Catholic Moral Theology in Dialogue*, Indiana, Fides, Notre Dame Press, 1976, 184–219.

Davidson, David, 'DIGNITY, Inc.: an alternative experience of church', in *New Blackfriars*, April 1987, 192–201.

Dignity Task Force on Sexual Ethics, 'Sexual ethics: experience, growth, challenge', in *Dignity USA*, December 1989, 1–16.

Ellingsten, Mark, 'Homosexuality and the Churches: a quest for the Nicene vision', in *Journal of Ecumenical Studies*, 1993, 354–71.

Fox, Matthew, 'The spiritual journey of the homosexual . . . and just about everybody else', in Nugent, R. (ed.), *A Challenge to Love: Gay and Lesbian Catholics in the Church*, New York, Crossroad, 1989, 189–204.

Friedman, Richard and Downey, Jennifer, 'Homosexuality', in *The New England Journal of Medicine*, 6 October 1994, 923–30.

Furnish, Victor Paul, 'Homosexual practices in biblical perspective', in Carey, John J. (ed.), *The Sexuality Debate in North American Churches, 1988–1995: Controversies, Unresolved Issues, Future Prospects*, Lewiston, New York, Edwin Mellen Press, 1995, 253–81.

Gallagher, Raphael, *Understanding the Homosexual*, Dublin, Veritas Publications, 1986.

Gallagher, Raphael, 'Homosexuality, discrimination and a Vatican document', in *Doctrine and Life*, 1992, 435–40.

Gill, Sean, 'Odd but not queer: English liberal protestant theologies of human sexuality and the gay paradigm', in *Theology and Sexuality*, September 1995, 48–57.

Jantzen, Grace M., 'Off the straight and narrow: toward a lesbian theology', in *Theology and Sexuality*, September 1995, 58–76.

Jeffrey, John, *'Permanent, Faithful, Stable': Christian Same-Sex Partnerships*, London, Affirming Catholicism, 1993.

Kelly, Kevin, 'Sexual ethics: experience, growth, challenge', in *The Month*, 1990, 368–73.

Kiely, Bartholomew, 'The pastoral care of homosexual persons', in *Briefing*, 6 March 1987, 75–80.

McManus, Jim, 'The messianic reason of theology in a lesbian and gay context: a statement of faith', in *Theology and Sexuality*, September 1996, 58–75.

Mahoney, Cardinal, 'Homosexuals in the military: three issues', in *Origins*, 25 February 1993, 621–3.

Markey, John, 'The "problem" of homosexuality', in *New Blackfriars*, 1994, 476–88.

Matzko, David McCarthy, 'Homosexuality and the practices of marriage', in *Modern Theology*, 1997, 371–97.

Moore, Gareth, 'Are homosexuals sick?', in *New Blackfriars*, January 1989, 15–19.

Nelson, James B., 'Homosexuality', in Macquarrie, John and Childress, James (eds), *A New Dictionary of Christian Ethics*, London, SCM, 1986, 271–4.

Nugent, Robert, 'Homosexuality and Magisterial teaching', in *Irish Theological Quarterly*, 1987, I, pp. 66–74.

Nugent, Robert, 'Homosexual rights and the Catholic community', in *Doctrine and Life*, 1994, 165–73.

Padgug, Robert A., 'Gay villain, gay hero: homosexuality and the social construction of AIDS', chapter 16 in Simmons, Christian and Peiss, Kathy with Padgug, Robert A. (eds), *Passion and Power: Sexuality in History*, Philadelphia, Temple University Press, 1989.

Peck, Chris, 'What is natural?' in *Modern Churchman*, 1989, 25–9.

Quinn, Archbishop John R., 'Toward an understanding of the letter "On the Pastoral Care of Homosexual Persons"', in *America*, 7 February 1987, 92–95 & 116.

Ramsey Colloquium, 'The homosexual movement: a response by the Ramsey Colloquium', in *The Month*, 1994, 260–5.

Rees, Elizabeth, 'What are we doing to our gay people?', in *Furrow*, 1990, 27–33.

Ritter, Kathleen and O'Neil, Craig, 'Moving through loss: the spiritual journey of gay men and lesbian women', in *Journal of Counselling and Development*, 1989, 9–15.

Roach, Archbishop, 'The rights of homosexual persons', in *Origins*, 7 November 1991, 356–7.

Rudy, Kathy, '"Where two or more are gathered": using gay communities as a model for Christian sexual ethics', in *Theology and Sexuality*, March 1996, 81–99.

Schuklenk, Udo, Stein, Edward, Kerin, Jacinta and Byne, William, 'The ethics of genetic research on sexual orientation', in *Hastings Center Report*, July/August 1997, 6–13.

Seubert, Xavier John, 'The sacramentality of metaphors: reflections on homosexuality', in *Cross Currents*, Spring 1991, 52–68.

Stuart, Elizabeth, 'Healing, not outing', in *The Tablet*, 17 December 1994.

Tuohey, John, 'The CDF and homosexuals: rewriting the moral tradition', in *America*, 12 September 1992, 136–8.

White, Leland J., 'Does the Bible speak about gays or same-sex orientation? A test case in biblical ethics I', in *Biblical Theology Bulletin*, 1995, 14–23.

Yip, Andrew, 'Gay Christian couples and blessing ceremonies', in *Theology and Sexuality*, March 1996, 100–17.

(7) ADDITIONAL WRITINGS QUOTED OR REFERRED TO IN THE BOOK

Anglican–Roman Catholic International Commission II, *Life in Christ: Morals, Communion and the Church*, London, Catholic Truth Society/Church House Publishing, 1994.

Bernardin, Cardinal Joseph, *Consistent Ethic of Life*, Kansas City, Sheed & Ward, 1988.

Berridge, Virginia, *AIDS in the UK: The Making of Policy, 1981–1994*, Oxford University Press, 1996.

Bouscaren, T. Lincoln and O'Connor, James I. (eds), *Canon Law Digest*, Milwaukee, Bruce, 1961 Supplement.

Burggraeve, Roger, 'Meaningful living and action: an ethical and educational pastoral model in Christian perspective', in *Louvain Studies*, 1988, 3–26 & 137–60.

Catholic Bishops' Conference of England and Wales, *The Common Good and the Catholic Church's Social Teaching* (1996).

Connors, Russell B., 'Thick and thin: an angle on Catholic moral teaching', in *Louvain Studies*, 1996, 336–55.

Davis, Charles, *Religion and the Making of Society: Essays in Social Theology*, Cambridge University Press, 1994.

Engel, Mary Potter, 'Historical theology and violence against women: unearthing a popular tradition of just battery', in Adams, Carol J. and Fortune, Marrie M. (eds), *Violence against Women and Children: A Christian Theological Sourcebook*, New York, Continuum, 1995, 242–62.

Fuchs, Josef, *Moral Demands and Personal Obligations*, Washington, Georgetown University Press, 1993.

Harris, Peter *et al.*, *On Human Life: An Examination of 'Humanae Vitae'*, London, Burns & Oates, 1968.

Keenan, James, 'Christian perspectives on the human body', in *Theological Studies*, 1994, 330–46.

Kelly, Kevin T., 'Conformity and dissent in the Church', in *The Way*, 1988, 87–101; *New Directions in Moral Theology*, London, Geoffrey Chapman, 1992: 'Moral theology in the parish', in *Priests and People*, 1994, 367–72; 'The Catechism and moral teaching: 10 tentative tips for readers', in *The Month*, July 1994, 266–9.

King, Ursula, review of Hawley, John Stratton (ed.), *Fundamentalism and Gender*, Oxford University Press, 1994, in *Theology and Sexuality*, vol. 3, 1995, 115–17.

Lash, Nicholas, *Believing Three Ways in God*, London, SCM, 1992.

McCormick, Richard, 'The search for truth in the Catholic context', in *America*, 8 November 1986, 276–81.

Merton, Thomas, *Conjectures of a Guilty Bystander*, London, Sheldon Press, 1977 edn.

National Catholic Reporter, Editorial, 15 September 1995, p. 24.

Noldin, H., *Summa Theologiae Moralis, vol III. De Sacramentis*, Barcelona, Herder, 27th edn, 1951.

Noonen, John, *Contraception: A History of Its Treatment by the Catholic Theologians and Canonists*, Cambridge, MA, Harvard University Press, 1965.

Pope John Paul II, *Veritatis Splendor* (1993); *Familiaris Consortio* (1981); *Sollicitudo Rei Socialis* (1987).

Pope Paul VI, *Humanae Vitae* (1968).

Pope Pius XI, *Casti Connubii* (1930).

Rahner, Karl, *Grace in Freedom*, Burns & Oates, London, 1969.

Rossetti, Stephen J., *Slayer of the Soul: Child Sexual Abuse and the Catholic Church*, Connecticut, Twenty-Third Publications, 1991.

Schillebeeckx, Edward, *God, the Future of Man*, London, Sheed & Ward, 1969.

Sherr, Lorraine, *Suicide Issues in a Cohort of HIV Positive Clinic Attenders: A Case Note Audit Study*, unpublished report prepared for the Health Education Authority, 1995.

Synod of Bishops, *Justice in the World*, Vatican Press, 1971.

Vatican II Pastoral Constitution, *The Church in the Modern World (Gaudium et Spes)* (1965).

Walker, Alice, *Possessing the Secret of Joy*, London, Vintage, 1993.

INDEX